SELF-THERAPIES FOR COMMON DISEASES

Li Hesheng

FOREIGN LANGUAGES PRESS BEIJING

First Edition 2001

Home Page:
http://www.flp.com.cn
E-mail Addresses:
info@flp.com.cn
sales@flp.com.cn

ISBN 7-119-02061-7

Published by Foreign Languages Press
24 Baiwanzhuang Road, Beijing 100037, China
Distributed by China International Book Trading Corporation
35 Chegongzhuang Xilu, Beijing 100044, China

Printed in the People's Republic of China

CONTENTS

PREPARATORY FORMS

Before you start a movement, you must prepare yourself for it.

Standing Form (1): Stand erect with feet together, arms hanging down naturally, and each palm touching the outside of the thigh, with the middle finger tips touching the acupoints of Fengshi (the points outside of the thighs where your middle finger tips touch when standing straight, your hands hanging down). Stand straight and look ahead, with your tongue touching the upper palate. Rest your weight equally on both feet. Free your mind of any thoughts, thus keeping both your body and mind in emptiness, calmness and relaxation. (See Fig. 1)

Standing Form (2): Standing with feet shoulder-width apart, arms hanging down naturally and each palm touching the outside of the thigh. Tough the acupoints of Fengshi with your middle finger tips. Look straight ahead, with your tongue touching the upper palate. Rest your weight on both feet. Free your mind of any thoughts, thus keeping both your body and mind in emptiness, calmness and relaxation. (See Fig. 2)

Standing Form (3): Stand with feet apart, the distance in between being a little wider than the shoulder-width. Turn toes slightly inward, with the arms hanging down naturally, each palm touching the outside of the thigh. Touch the acupoints of Fengshi with your middle finger tips. Bend your knees slightly, with the kneecaps in a line vertically above the toes. Look straight ahead, with your tongue touching the upper palate. Rest your weight equally on both feet. (See Fig. 3)

Sitting Form: Sit erect on a chair, with your feet shoulder-width apart. Keep the thighs at a right angle to the calves, the trunk upright, the whole body relaxed, and the chin pulled in slightly (as shown in Fig. 4).

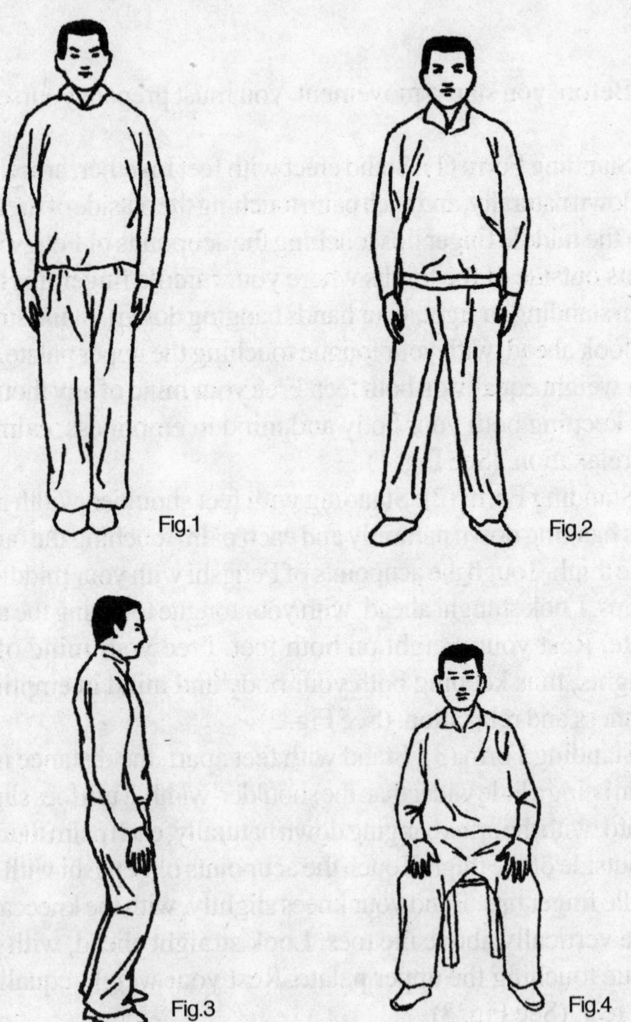

MEASUREMENT OF THE LOCATION OF ACUPOINTS

Form a ring with your thumb and your middle finger. Take the length between the two ends of the transverse lines of the middle section of the middle finger as one cun (the length of the unit varies according to the height of different individuals, as shown in Fig. 5), and one tenth of this cun as one fen.

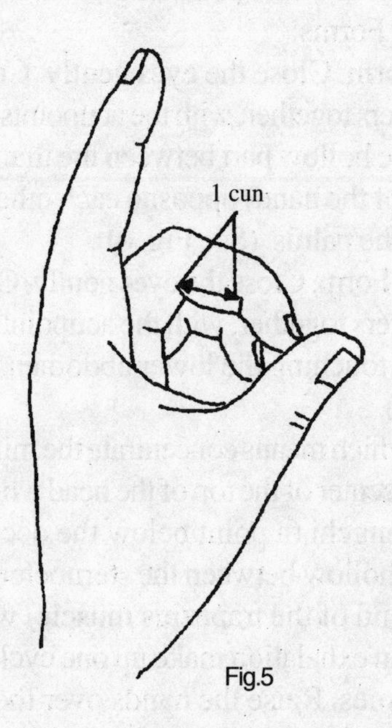

Fig.5

CHAPTER I THE CEREBRAL AND CARDIO VASCULAR SYSTEM

1. The Exercise for Invigorating the Function of the Brain and Developing Intelligence

Self-Therapy Indication: This exercise can prevent cerebral vascularsclerosis, and invigorate memory and the function of the brain.

It can be done in either a standing or sitting form.

Preparatory Forms:

1) Sitting form. Close the eyes gently. Connect the thumbs and the forefingers together, with the acupoints of Hegu (a point in the middle of the hollow part between the thumb and the forefinger at the back of the hand) opposite each other. Touch the lower abdomen with the palms. (See Fig. 6)

2) Standing Form. Close the eyes gently. Connect the thumbs and the forefingers together, with the acupoints of Hegu opposite each other, and touching the lower abdomen with the palms (as shown in Fig. 7).

Visualise (which means concentrate the mind on) the acupoint of Baihui at the center of the top of the head while inhaling and the acupoints of Fengchi (a point below the occipital bones in the cervical part, a hollow between the sternocleidomastoid muscle and the upper end of the trapezius muscle) while exhaling. An inhalation and an exhalation make up one cycle, which should be repeated 108 times. Raise the hands over the sides of the head (as shown in Fig. 8 and Fig. 9). Make 108 circles first upward and then backward with hands. Then make another 108 circles

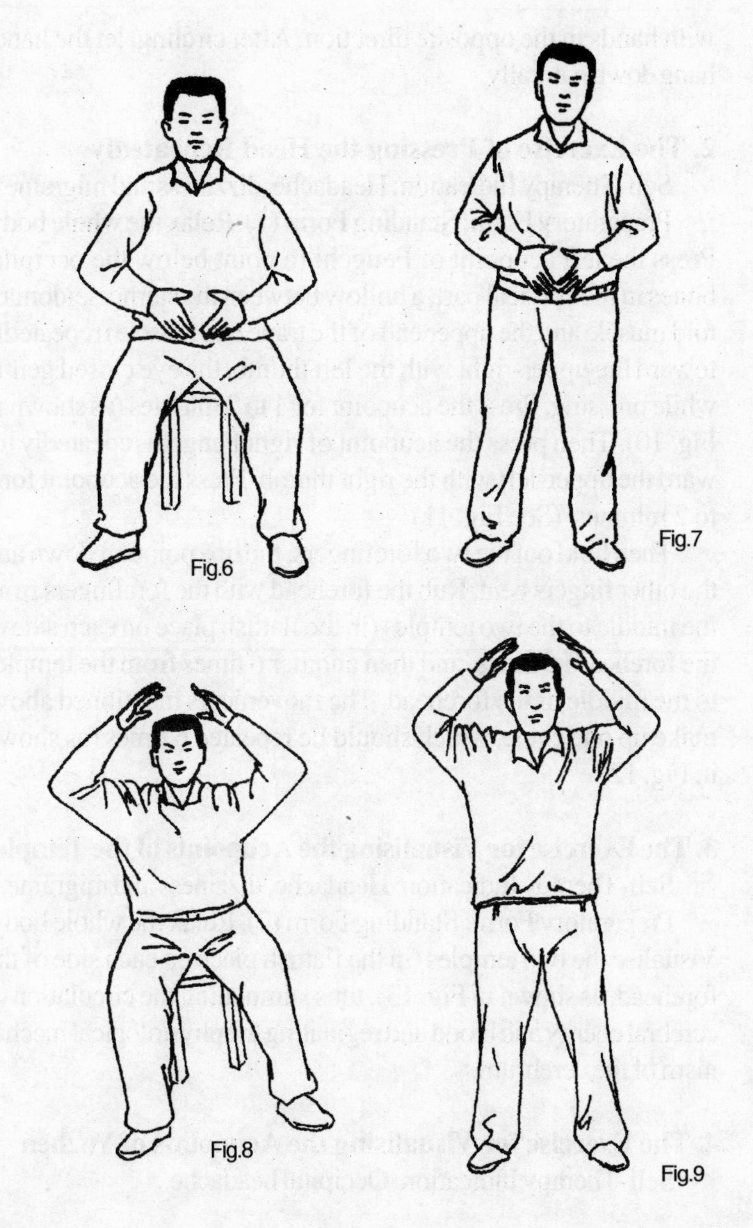

Fig.6 Fig.7 Fig.8 Fig.9

with hands in the opposite direction. After circling, let the hands hang down naturally.

2. The Exercise of Pressing the Head Repeatedly

Self-Therapy Indication: Headache, dizziness and migraine.

Preparatory Form: Standing Form (1). Relax the whole body. Press the left acupoint of Fengchi (a point below the occipital bones in the cervical part, a hollow between the sternocleidomastoid muscle and the upper end of the trapezius muscle) repeatedly toward the upper-right with the left thumb, the eye closed gently while pressing. Press the acupoint for 1 to 2 minutes (as shown in Fig. 10). Then press the acupoint of right Fengchi repeatedly toward the upper-left with the right thumb. Press the acupoint for 1 to 2 minutes. (See Fig. 11)

Then hold out the two forefingers, the tips pointing down and the other fingers bent. Rub the forehead with the forefingers from the middle to the two temples (in the flattish place on each side of the forehead) 6 times, and then another 6 times from the temples to the middle of the forehead. The movements mentioned above make up one cycle, which should be repeated 6 times (as shown in Fig. 12).

3. The Exercise for Visualising the Acupoints of the Temples

Self-Therapy Indication: Headache, dizziness and migraine.

Preparatory Form: Standing Form (2). Relax the whole body. Visualise the two temples (in the flattish place on each side of the forehead, as shown in Fig. 13), thus stimulating the circulation of cerebral energy and blood and regulating the physiological mechanism of the cerebrum.

4. The Exercise for Visualising the Acupoints of Yuzhen

Self-Therapy Indication: Occipital headache.

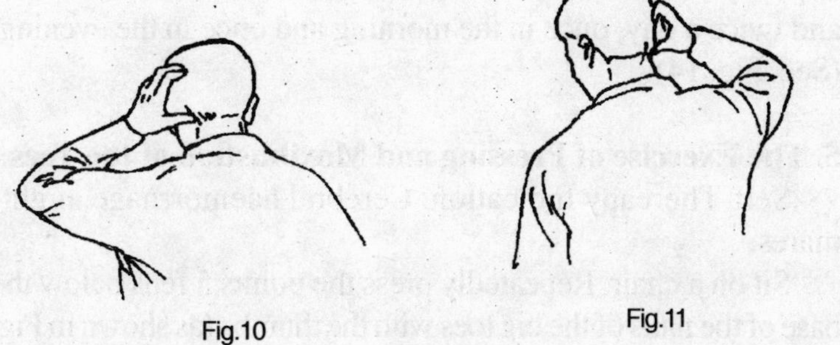

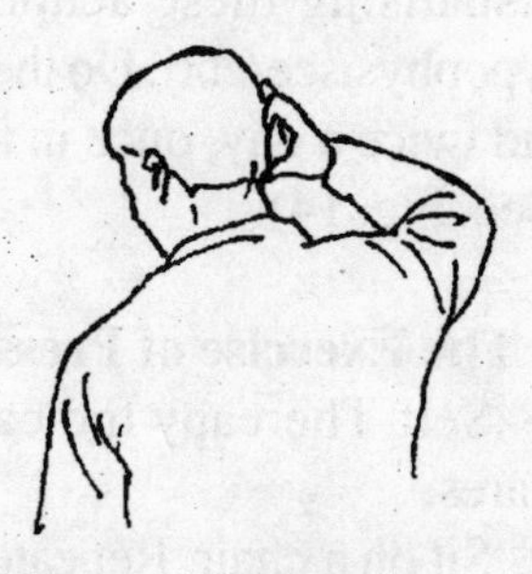

Fig.10

Fig.11

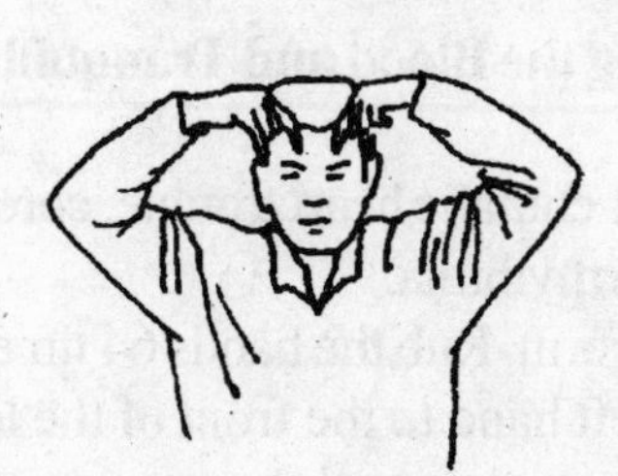

Fig.12

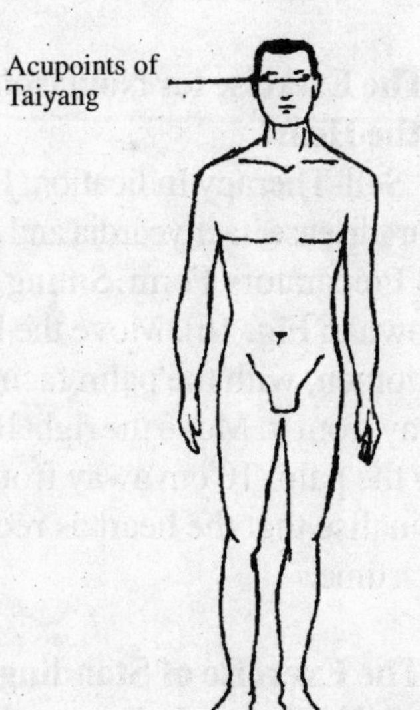

Fig.13

Preparatory Form: Standing Form (2). Relax the whole body, visualising the acupoints of Yuzhen at the back of the head. Visualising these acupoints can increase the secretion of hypophysiscerebri. Do the exercise for 20 minutes each session and twice a day, once in the morning and once in the evening. (See Fig. 14)

5. The Exercise of Pressing and Moxibustion of the Toes

Self-Thereapy Indication: Cerebral haemorrhage, nightmares.

Sit on a chair. Repeatedly press the points 5 fens below the base of the nails of the big toes with the thumbs (as shown in Fig. 15). Press the points repeatedly until you feel sore and numb in the area. Then administer moxibustion at each point with a moxaroll for 10 minutes.

6. The Exercise for Nourishing the Blood and Tranquillising the Heart

Self-Therapy Indication: Rheumatic heart trouble, coronary heart disease, tachycardia and arrhythmia.

Preparatory Form: Sitting Form. Rub the hands 64 times (as shown in Fig. 16). Move the left hand to the front of the lower abdomen, with the palm facing the lower abdomen and 10 cm away from it. Move the right hand to the front of the heart, keeping the palm 10 cm away from the chest (as shown in Fig. 17). Visualise that the heart as red. Do the exercise for 10 minutes each time.

7. The Exercise of Standing to Discharge Rheumatism

Self-Therapy Indication: Rheumatic heart trouble and rheumatoid arthritis.

Preparatory Form: Standing Form (2). Relax the whole body.

Stretch the arms out from the left and right sides, with the arms at an angle of 90 degrees to each other, and the palms facing forward. Hold out the fingers naturally, keeping your mind on the fingers (as shown in Fig. 18). Do the exercise twice daily and each time

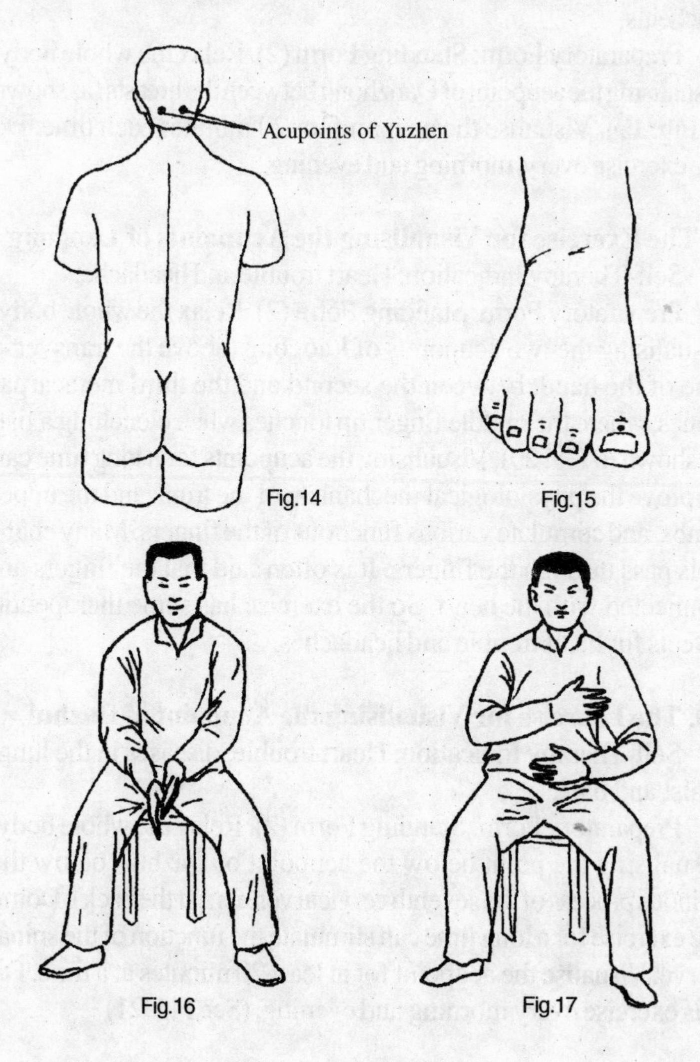

Fig.14

Fig.15

Fig.16

Fig.17

for 20 minutes.

8. The Exercise for Visualising the Acupoint of Danzhong

Self-Therapy Indication: Myocarditis, pneumonia, pharynx and tracheitis.

Preparatory Form: Standing Form (2). Relax the whole body, visualising the acupoint of Danzhong between the breasts (as shown in Fig. 19). Visualise the acupoint for 20 minutes each time. Do the exercise every morning and evening.

9. The Exercise for Visualising the Acupoints of Laogong

Self-Therapy Indication: Heart trouble and headache.

Preparatory Form: Standing Form (2). Relax the whole body, visualising the two acupoints of Laogong (above the transverse line of the hand, between the second and the third metacarpal bones, where the middle finger tip touches when clenching a fist, as shown in Fig. 20). Visualising the acupoints for a long time can improve the physiological mechanism of the trunk and the upper limbs, and stimulate various functions of the fingers. Many channels pass through the fingers. It is often said that the fingers are connected with the heart. So the exercise has some therapeutic effects for heart trouble and headaches.

10. The Exercise for Visualising the Acupoint of Dazhui

Self-Therapy Indication: Heart trouble, diseases in the lung, waist and back.

Preparatory Form: Standing Form (2). Relax the whole body, visualising the point below the acupoint of Dazhui (below the spinous process of the seventh cervical vertebra at the back). Doing the exercise for a long time can stimulate the function of the spinal nerve. Visualise the acupoint for at least 20 minutes at a time. Do this exercise every morning and evening. (See Fig. 21)

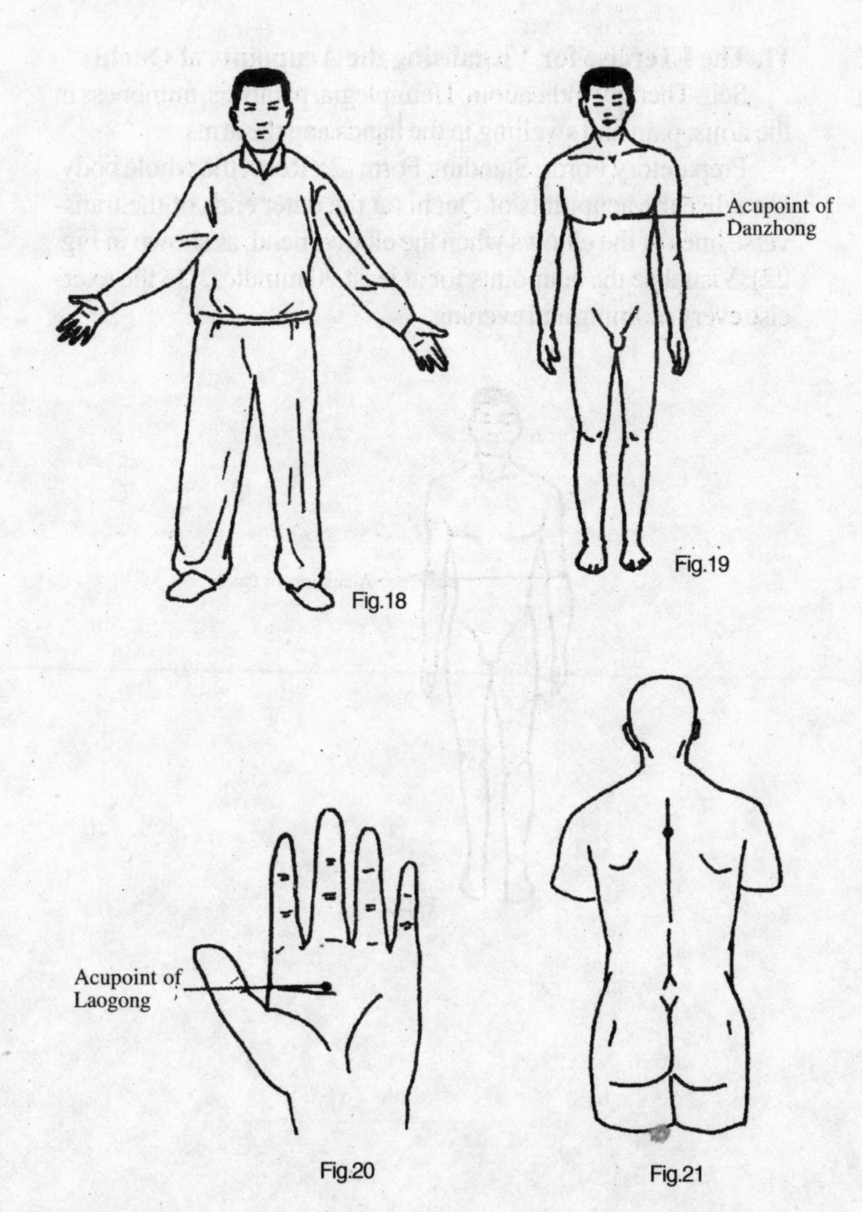

Fig.18

Fig.19

Fig.20

Fig.21

11. The Exercise for Visualising the Acupoints of Quchi

Self-Therapy Indicatioin: Hemiplegia, paralysis, numbness in the arms, pain and swelling in the hands and the arms.

Preparetory Form: Standing Form (2). Relax the whole body. Visualise the acupoints of Quchi (at the outer ends of the transverse lines of the elbows when the elbows bend, as shown in Fig. 22). Visualise the acupoints for at least 20 minutes. Do the exercise every morning and evening.

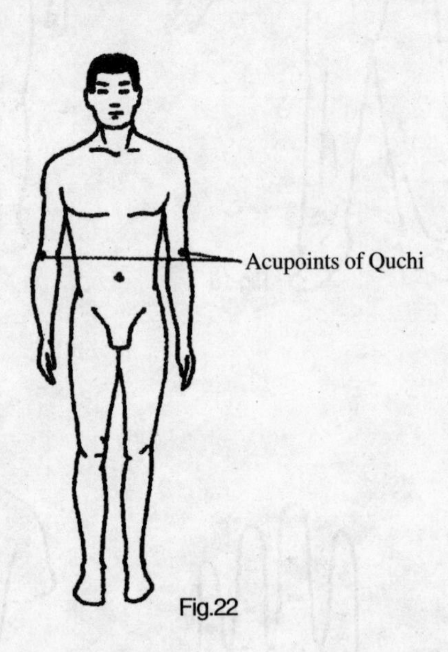

Fig.22

CHAPTER II HYPERTENSION AND HYPOTENSION

1. The Exercise for Lowering Hypertension

Self-Therapy Indication: This exercise has an especially good effects on hypertension. It also has an effect on insubstantial *Yin* and over flourishing *Yang*, and the deficiency of *Yin* and *Yang*.

Preparatory Forms:

1) Standing Form (2). Close the eyes gently. Relax the arms, moving the hands to the front of the lower abdomen, with the palms facing up and the two middle fingers touching each other. Imagine it is drizzling, rainwater flowing slowly from the top of the head down the face, then down the chest and the back. Now you should feel cool and refreshed all over. Stand this way for 10 to 20 minutes at a time, and then imagine that the rain stops and let your hands hang down naturally. (See Fig. 23)

2) Sitting Form. Put the hands beside the thighs with each hand 10 cm away from each thigh. Bend the elbows slightly, with the palms facing down, and fingers pointing forward. Close your eyes gently. Imagine that the two acupoints of Laogong above the transverse line (between the seconde and the third metacarpal bones where the middle finger touches when clenching a fist, as shown in Fig. 20) are connected with the two acupoints of Yongquan (in the hollow in the center of the sole when the toes bend, as shown Fig. 25). Sit still this way for 20 minutes each session.(See Fig. 24)

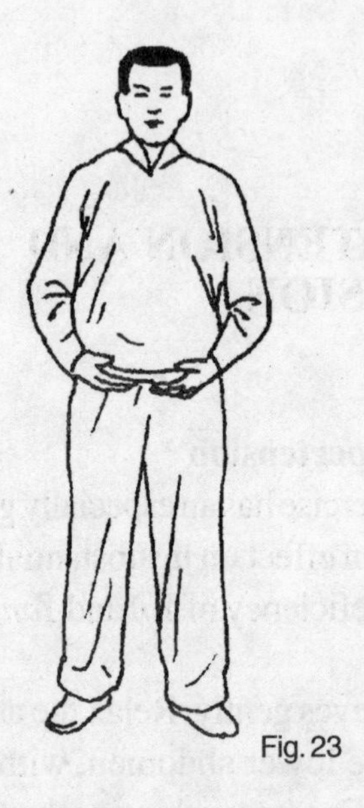

Fig. 23

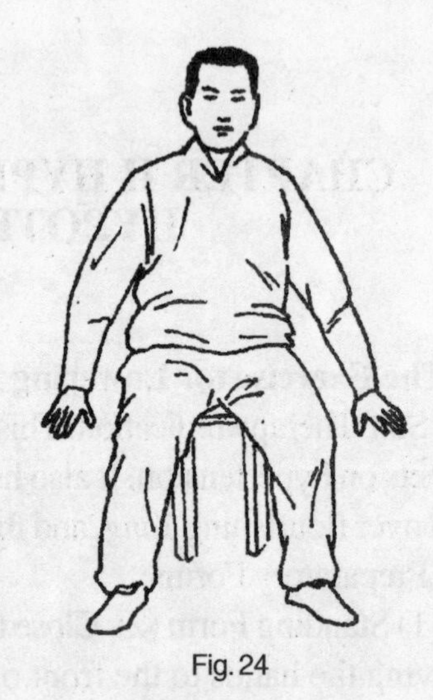

Fig. 24

2. The Exercise for Visualising the Acupoints of Yongquan

Self-Therapy Indication: Hypertension, and the deficiency of the kidneys.

Preparatory Form: Standing Form (2). Relax the whole body, visualising the acupoints of Yongquan (in the hollow in the center of the sole when the toes bend, as shown in Fig. 25). Visualising the acupoints for a long time can make you relaxed, thus discharging pathogenic air from your body, and stimulating the circulation of the vital energy and blood through your body.

3. The Exercise for Curing Hypotension

Self-Therapy Indication: Doing this exercise regularly can help overcome low blood pressure.

Preparatory Forms:

1) Sitting form. Close the eyes gently. Raise the hands slowly, bending at the elbows. Direct the palms toward the breasts, keep-

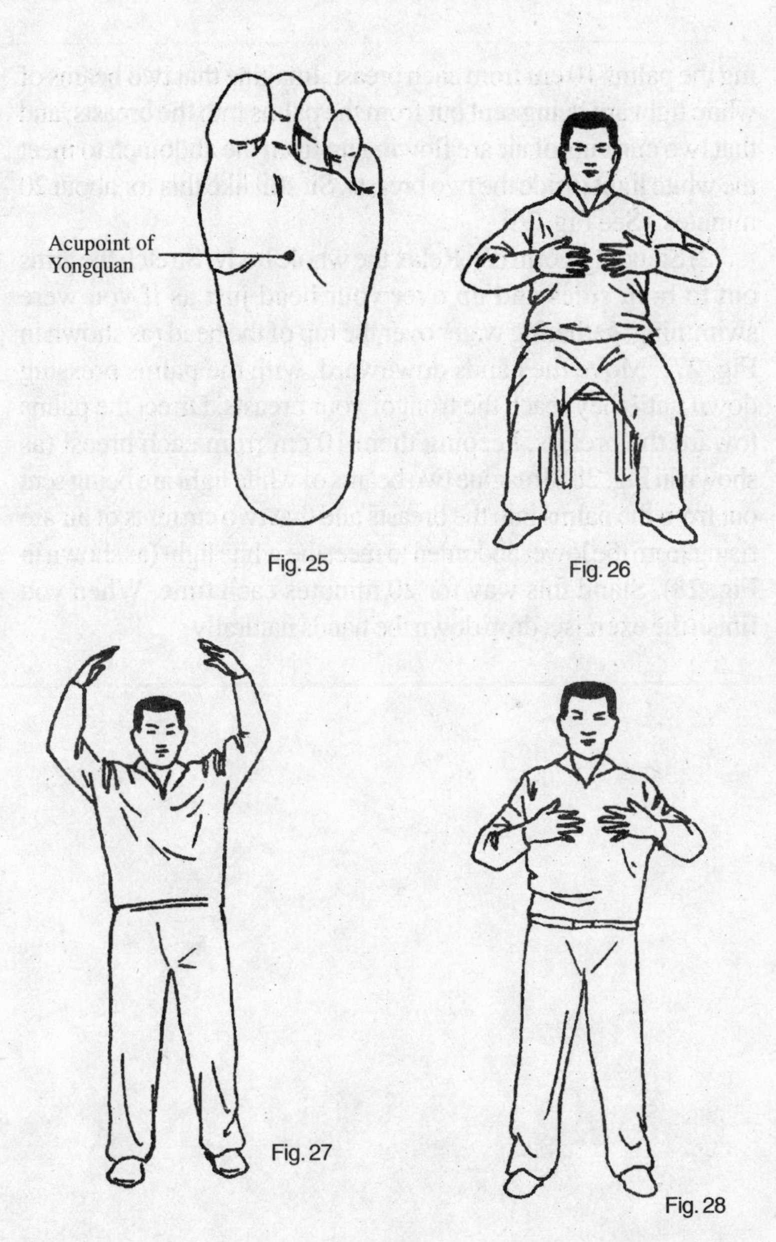

Fig. 25

Fig. 26

Fig. 27

Fig. 28

ing the palms 10 cm from each breast. Imagine that two beams of white light are being sent out from the palms into the breasts, and that two currents of air are flowing up from the abdomen to meet the white light inside the two breasts. Sit still like this for about 20 minutes. (See Fig. 26)

2) Standing Form (2). Relax the whole body. Stretch the arms out to both sides and up over your head just as if you were swimming, gathering water over the top of the head (as shown in Fig. 27). Move the hands downward, with the palms pressing down until they reach the front of your breasts. Direct the palms toward the breasts, keeping them 10 cm from each breast (as shown in Fig. 28). Imagine two beams of white light are being sent out from the palms into the breasts and that two currents of air are rising from the lower abdomen to meet the white light (as shown in Fig. 28). Stand this way for 20 minutes each time. When you finish the exercise, drop down the hands naturally.

CHAPTER III THE NERVOUS SYSTEM

1. The Exercise for Relaying and Entering into Quiescence

Self-Therapy Indication: This exercise can recuperate the nerves, cure neurathenia, fidgeting, stuffy chest, tracheitis, hypertension and insomnia. It can be done in either standing, sitting or lying forms.

Preparatory Forms:

1) Sitting Form. Relax the whole body, putting the hands on the thighs and closing the eyes gently (as shown in Fig. 29).

2) Standing Form (2). Relax the whole body, closing the eyes gently (as shown in Fig. 30).

3) Lying Form: Relax the whole body. Lie on your back, resting your head on a pillow of moderate height. Keep the feet shoulder-width apart. Put the hands near the outside of the thighs, with palms facing down and the eyes closed. (See Fig. 31)

Keep your mind on relaxing the top of your head, ears, shoulders, upper arms, forearms, hands and finger tips, respectively. Then again relax the top of the head, then the face, the neck and the throat, the chest, the abdomen, the perineum, the two thights, the knees, the shanks, the insteps, the big toes, the second toes, the third toes, the fourth toes, the little toes, and the soles, respectively. Imagine your feet to be in warm water. (In summer, imagine them to be in cold water). Finally, silently repeat the phrase "relax the entire body" 3 times.

2. The Exercise for Channelling the Qi Through the Chest

The Qi is referred to as the refined nutritive substance flowing within the body.

Self-Therapy Indication: Stuffy chest, difficulty in breathing.

Preparatory Form: Standing Form (2): Relax the whole body, closing the eyes gently. Bend the knees slightly and stand still for 5 minutes. Then imagine that two streams are flowing down from the nipples to the navel. Continue to imagine this for 5 minutes. (See Fig. 32)

3. The Exercise for Visualising the Acupoint of Baihui

Self-Therapy Indication: Headache and dizziness. This exercise can promote the function of memory and the ability to reason.

Preparatory Form: Standing Form (2). Relax the whole body. Visualise the acupoint of Baihui (at which the middle line parting the hair intersects the line from the ears' apex, as shown in Fig. 33). Visualising this acupoint for a long time can strengthen the physiological function of the cerebrum, keeping the cerebrum in a relatively inhibited state and stimulating blood and vital energy circulation in the cerebrum. (See Fig. 33)

4. The Exercise of Pressing the Acupoints of Tianxin

Self-Therapy Indication: High heat coma.

Knead with the thumbs 36 times the acupoints of Little Tianxin (at the intersection of big thenar eminence and small thenar eminence in the two palms, as shown in Fig. 34). Exert force while kneading. (See Fig. 35)

5. The Exercise for Channelling the Qi to Cure Insomnia

Self-Therapy Indication: Insomnia.

This exercise can be done either in a sitting form or a lying form. It is better for those who suffer from serious insomnia to do the exercise in a laying form.

Preparatory Forms:

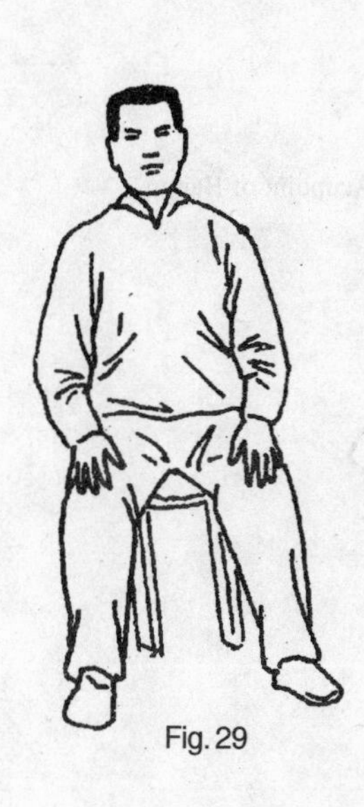

Fig. 29

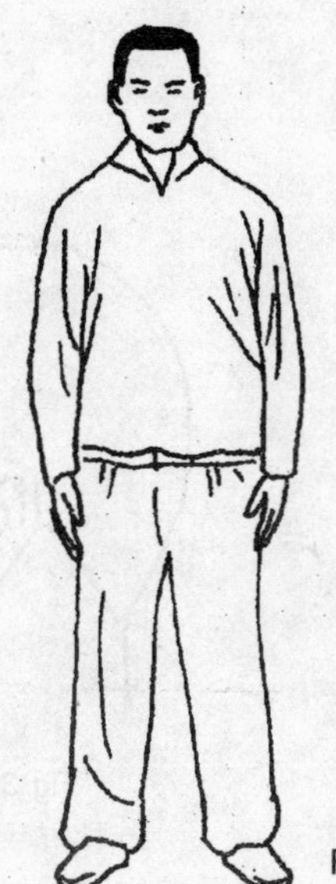

Fig. 30

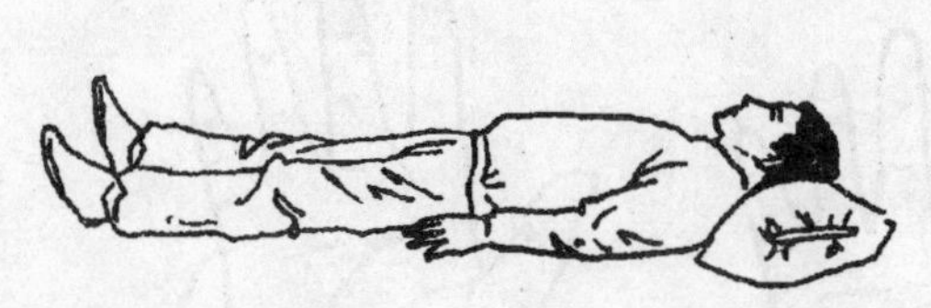

Fig. 31

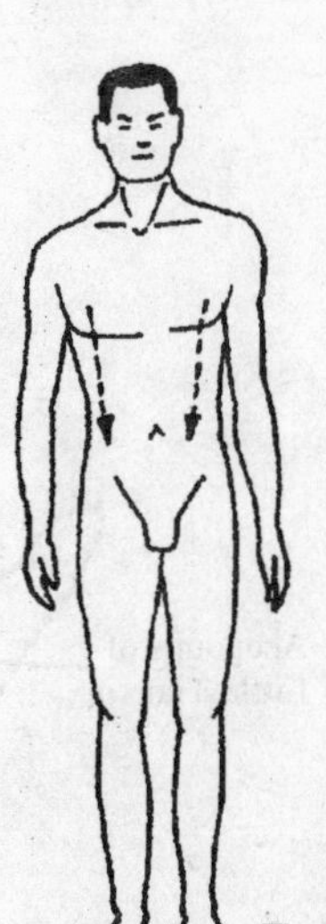

Fig. 32

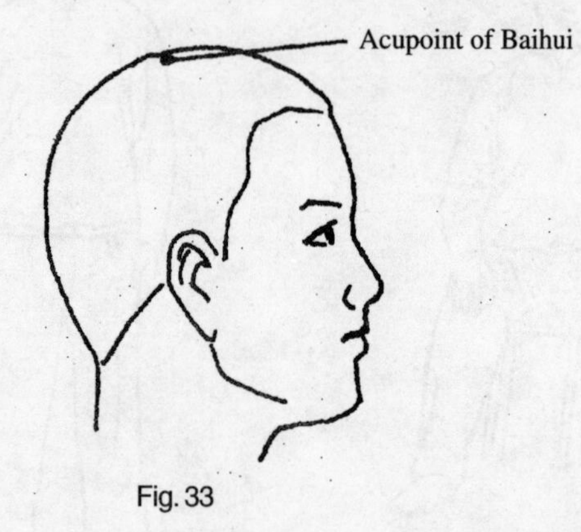

Fig. 33

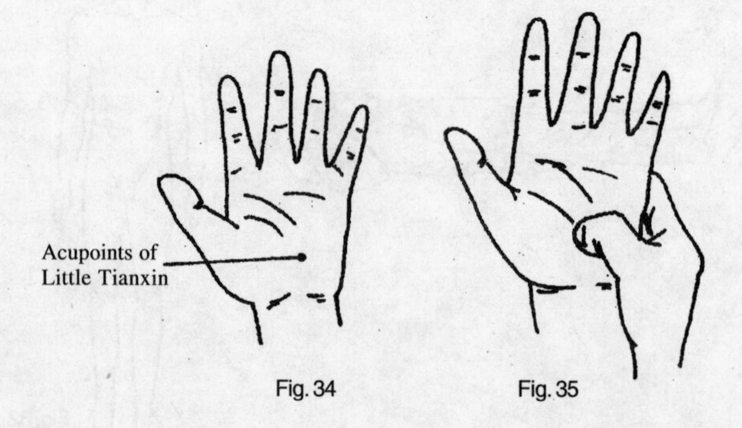

Fig. 34

Fig. 35

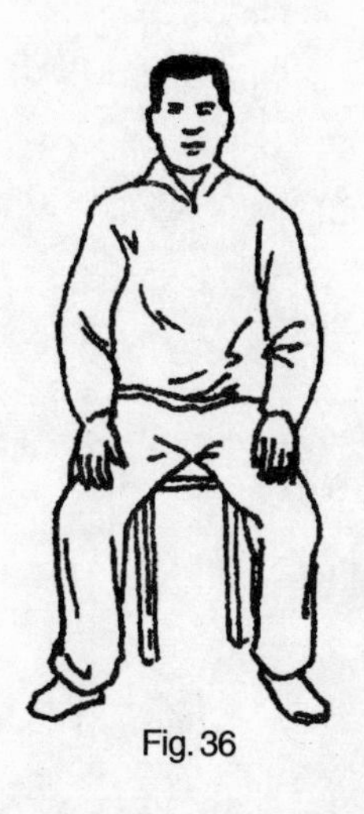
Fig. 36

1) Sitting Form. Relax the whole body (as shown in Fig. 36). Close the eyes gently, sitting still for 2 or 3 minutes. Visualise the acupoint of Baihui at the top of the head for one minute. Then visualise the acupoints of Jianjing, Danzhong, the Middle Dantian, Huiyin, Xuehai (in the inner side of thighs), Yinlingquan, Sanyinjiao, Zhaohai (in the inner ankles), Yongquan, the big toes, the second toes, the third toes, the fourth toes, the little toes, and then the acupoints of Yongquan. Imagine soaking the two acupoints of Yongquan in water. Then visualise the acupoints Shenmai in the outer ankles, Xuanzhong, Yanglingquan, Fengshi, Huantiao, Huiyin, Mingmen, the Middle Dantian, Xuehai, Yinlingquan, Sanyinjiao, Zhaohai, and Yongquan. Imagine soaking the acupoints of Yongquan in water. What has been mentioned above is one cycle (as shown in Fig. 37 and Fig. 38). Those who suffer from the most serious insomnia should be able to go to sleep after repeating the exercise 3 times.

2) Lying Form. Either lying on the back or on the side will do. Visualise the acupoints mentioned above each for half a minute or one minute. Don't do it in a hurry. If the patient is seriously ill, his relative can sit by him and recite the names of the acupoints in a low voice. The patient's imagination should follow the reciting. Recite the acupoints in a mild, even and moderate tune. (See Fig. 39 and Fig. 40)

6. The Exercise of Sitting Cross-Legged to Channel the Qi

Self-Therapy Indication: Sleep-addiction, and lethargy.

Sit cross-legged naturally, keeping the trunk straight and the

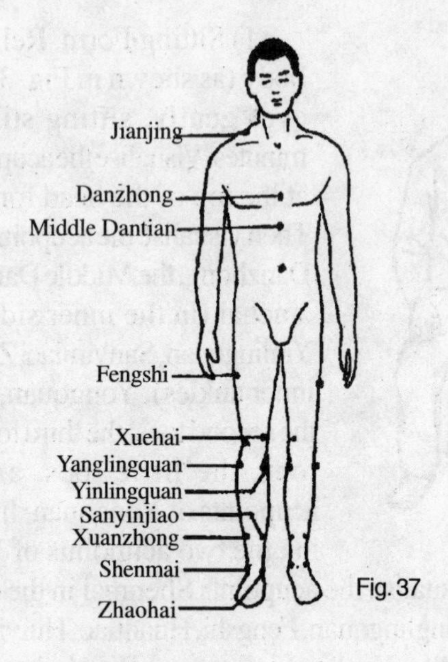
Jianjing
Danzhong
Middle Dantian
Fengshi
Xuehai
Yanglingquan
Yinlingquan
Sanyinjiao
Xuanzhong
Shenmai
Zhaohai
Fig. 37

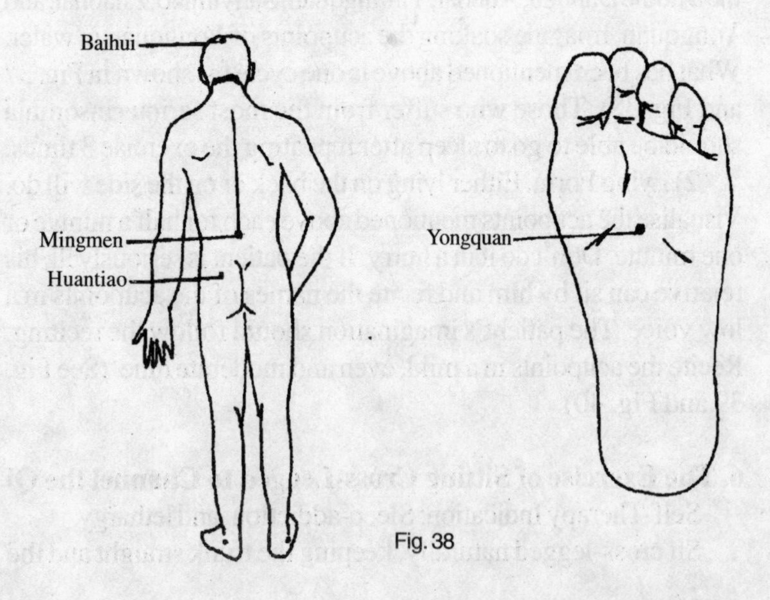
Baihui
Mingmen
Huantiao
Yongquan
Fig. 38

whole body relaxed. Hold the right foot with the left hand and the left foot with the right hand, pulling the feet hard to the left and right sides 6 times (as shown in Fig. 41). Then cross the arms and extend them past the inside of the thighs to hold the feet. Hold the left foot with the left hand and the right foot with the right hand. Pull the feet hard backward 6 times (as shown in Fig. 42).

7. The Exercise of Clenching Fists to Channel the Qi

Self-Therapy Indication: Nightmare.

Clench the fists, with the thumbs bent towards the centre of

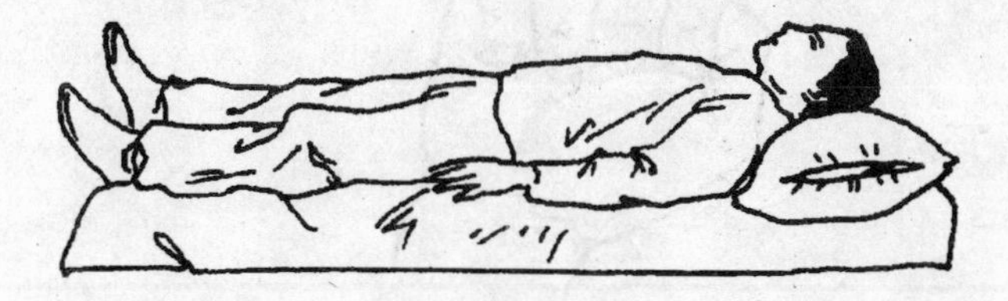

Fig. 39

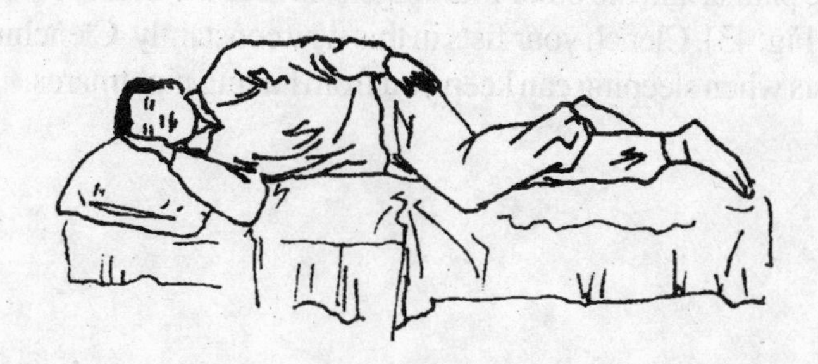

Fig. 40

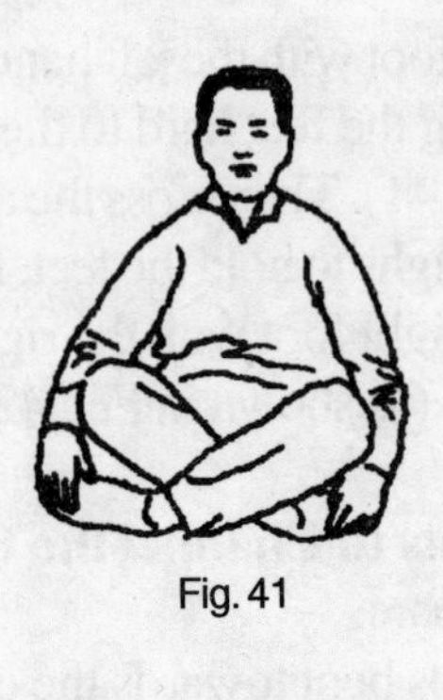

Fig. 41

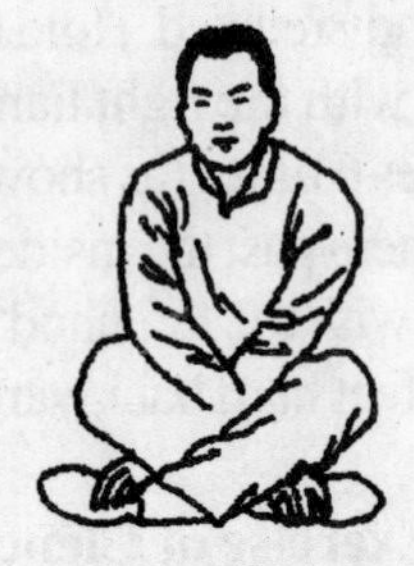

Fig. 42

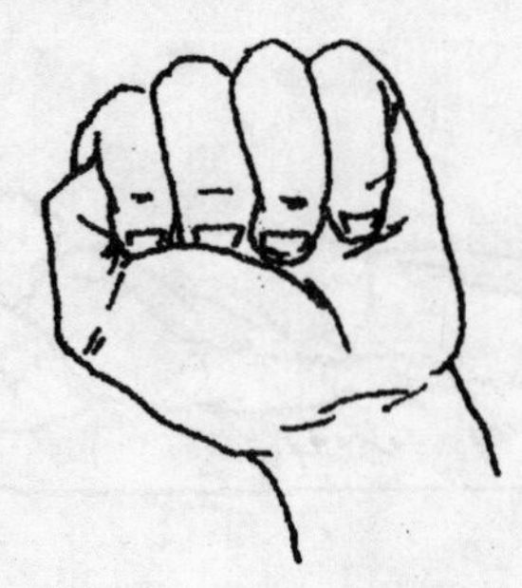

Fig. 43

the palms, and the other four fingers outside the thumb (as shown in Fig. 43). Clench your fists in this way constantly. Clenching the fists when sleeping can keep you from having nightmares.

CHAPTER IV THE KIDNEY AND THE INTERNAL SECRETION SYSTEM

1. The Exercise for Curing Diabetes

Self-Therapy Indication: Diabetes, pain in the abdomen.

Preparatory Form: Standing Form (1). Relax the shoulders and elbows. Stretch the arms out to the sides, left and right, and then move them in an arc until the hands close in front of the chest (as shown in Fig. 44).

Stretch the arms forward, keeping them above the navel (as shown in Fig. 45). Turn the left palm up, drawing the left elbow backward. Move the hands along the left ribs, pressing the left ribs with the right forearm (as shown in Fig. 46). Turn the thumbs up and turn the waist, moving the hands to the front of the body (as shown in Fig. 47). Turn the right palm up, drawing the right elbow backward. Move the hands along the right ribs until the left forearm press the right ribs (as shown in Fig. 48). Turn the thumbs up and turn the waist, moving the hands in front of you again (as shown in Fig. 49). The movements mentioned above make up one cycle, which should be repeated 24 times.

Closing Form: Keep the hands close in front of the chest (as shown in Fig. 50). Separate the little fingers, the fourth fingers, the middle fingers, the forefingers and the thumbs, respectively. Put the hands down naturally, returning to Standing Form (1).

Press 36 times the acupoint of Chengjiang in the middle point of the chin with the left forefinger. (See Fig. 51)

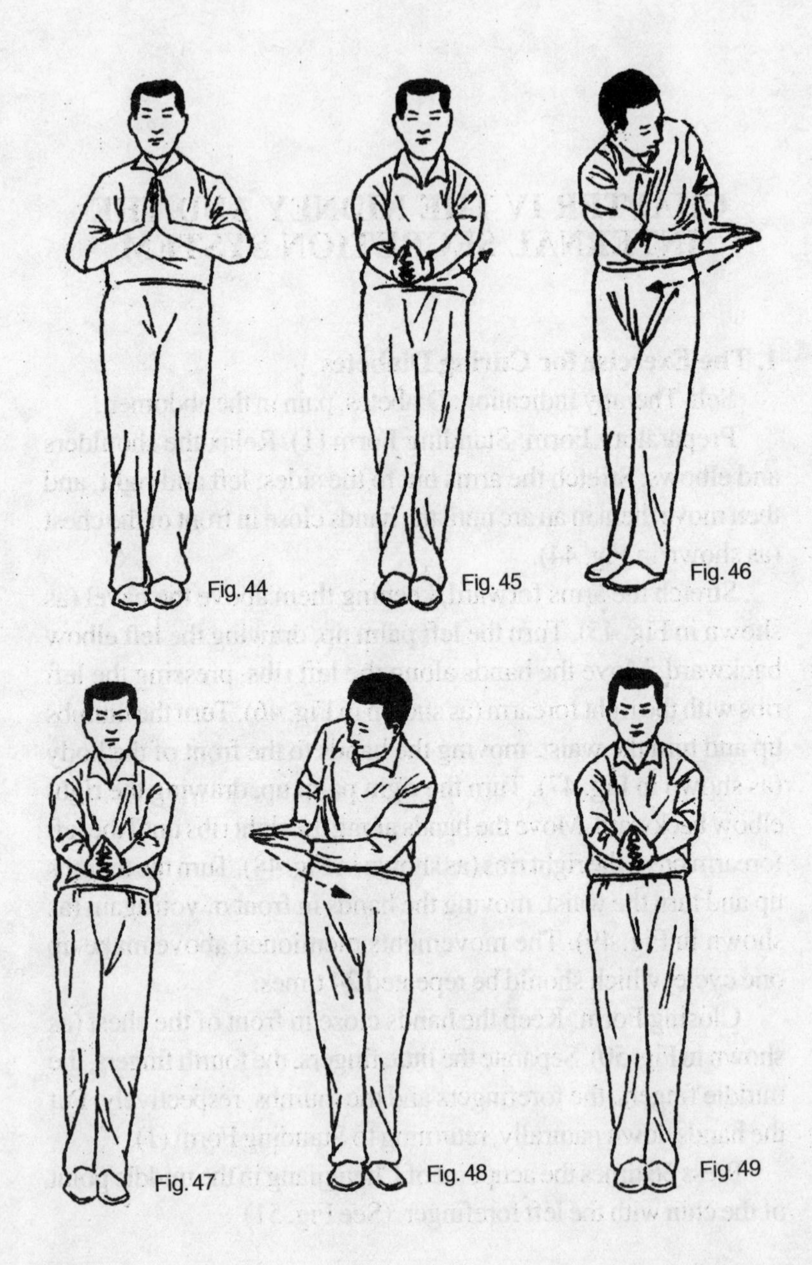

Fig. 44 Fig. 45 Fig. 46

Fig. 47 Fig. 48 Fig. 49

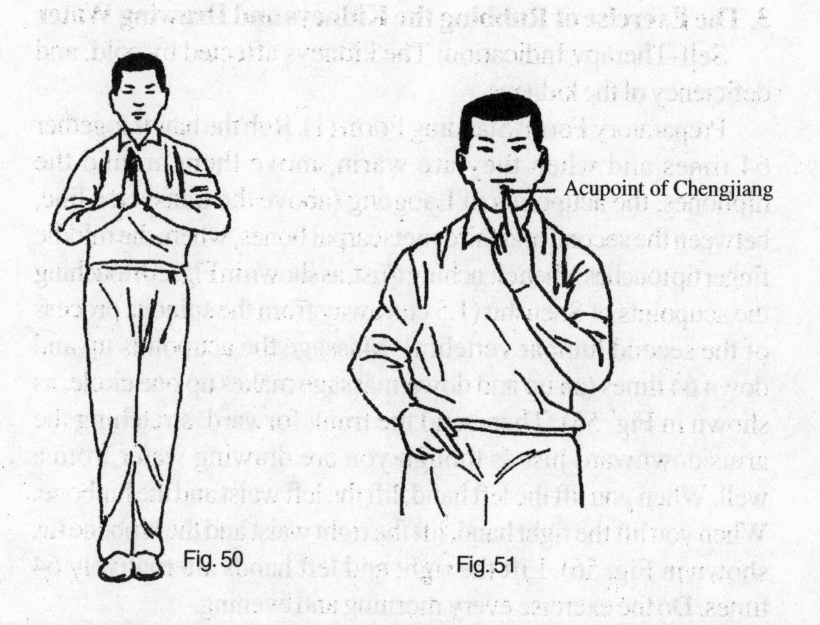

Fig. 50 Fig. 51

2. The Exercise for Channelling Qi by Horizontally Circling the Arms

Self-Therapy Indication: Endocrinopathy.

Preparatory Form: Standing Form (1). Keep the hands close in front of the body, the arms straight and the thumbs upright (as shown in Fig. 52). Turn the left palm up, pulling the left elbow backward. Make a horizontal circle to the left with the hands until the right forearm presses the left ribs. (See Fig. 53)

Turn the thumbs up and turn the hands with the waist in front of the trunk, and the arms straight. Turn the right palm up, pulling the right elbow backward. Make a circle to the right with the hands until the left forearm presses the right ribs (as shown in Fig. 54). The left-arc and the right-arc movements make up one cycle, which should be repeated 12 times.

3. The Exercise of Rubbing the Kidneys and Drawing Water

Self-Therapy Indication: The kidneys affected by cold, and deficiency of the kidneys.

Preparatory Form: Standing Form (1). Rub the hands together 64 times and when they are warm, move them around the hiphones, the acupoints of Laogong (above the transverse line, between the second and third metacarpal bones, where the middle finger tip touches when clenching a fist, as shown in Fig. 20) touching the acupoints of Shenshu (1.5 cun away from the spinous process of the second lumbar vertebra). Massage the acupoints up and down 64 times (an up and down massage makes up one circle, as shown in Fig. 55). Then bend the trunk forward, stretching the arms downward just as though you are drawing water from a well. When you lift the left hand, lift the left waist and the hipbone. When you lift the right hand, lift the right waist and the hipbone (as shown in Fig. 56). Lift the right and left hands alternatively 64 times. Do the exercise every morning and evening.

4. The Exercise for Visualising the Acupoint of Mingmen

Self-Therapy Indication: Regulating the function of the adrenal gland and raising the body temperature.

Preparatory Form: Standing Form (2). Relax the whole body, visualising the acupoint of Mingmen (in the hollow below the spinous process of the second lumbar vertebra). This point lies where the adrenal gland is located. Visualise the acupoint for 20 minutes. Do the exercise twice a day. (See Fig. 57)

5. The Exercise for Strengthening the Kidneys

Self-Therapy Indication: This exercise can strengthen the kidneys and compensate for debility of the kidneys.

Preparatory Form: Standing Form (2). Relax the whole body. Stretch your arms out to the left and right and raise them as high as

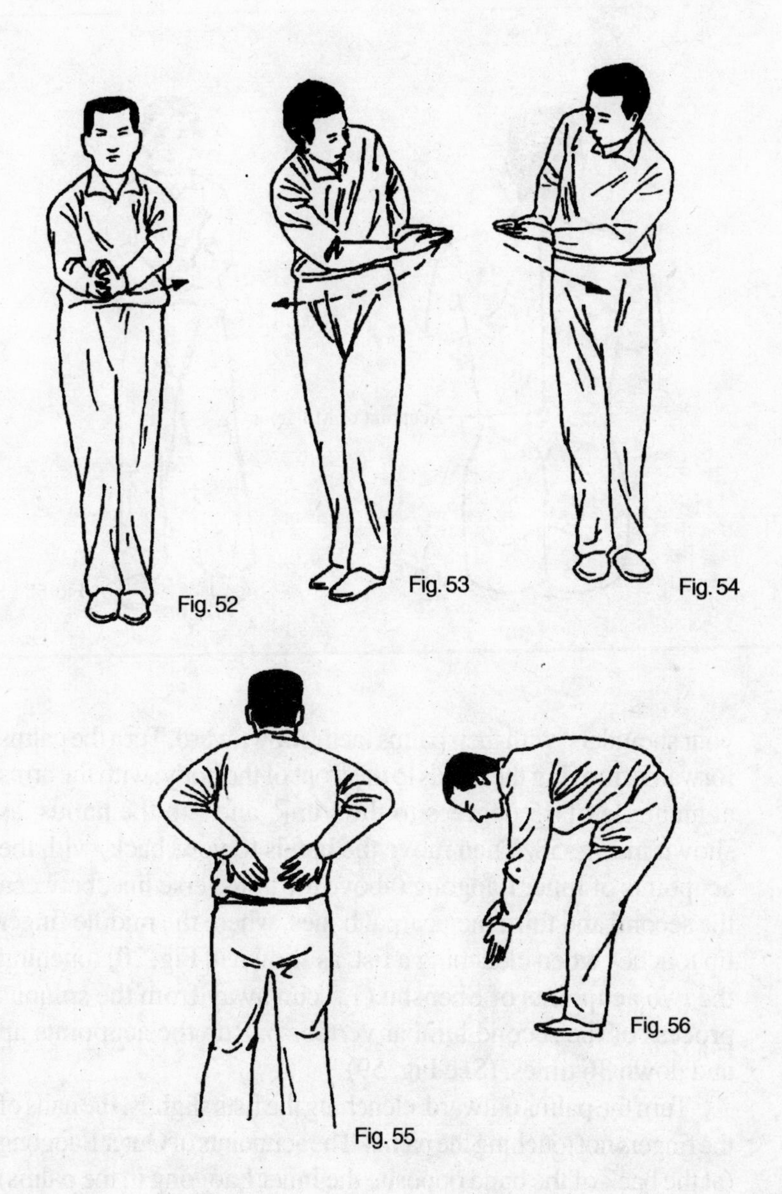
Fig. 52
Fig. 53
Fig. 54
Fig. 55
Fig. 56

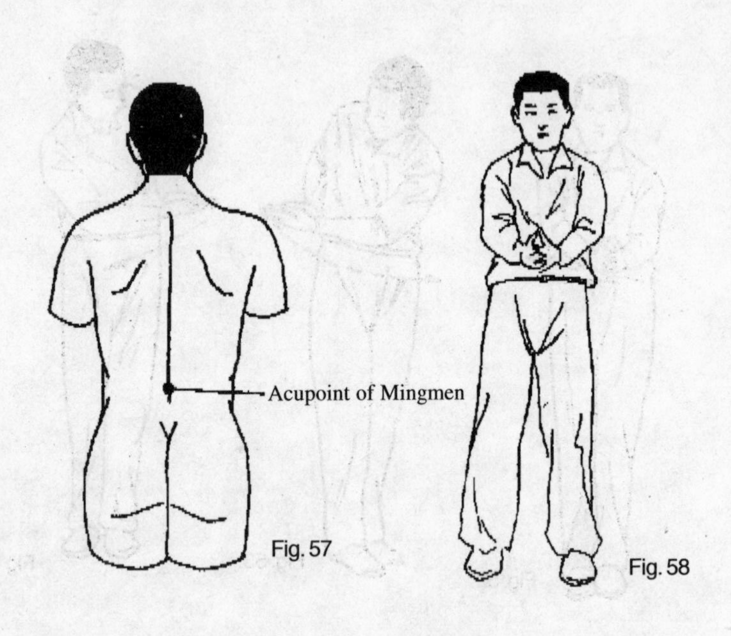

Fig. 57

Fig. 58

your shoulders, with their palms facing downward. Turn the palms forwards, moving the hands to the front of the body, with the arms at an angle of 45 degrees to the trunk, and rub the hands, as shown in Fig. 58. Then move the hands to your back, with the acupoints of Inner Laogong (above the transverse line, between the second and third metacarpal bones, where the middle finger tip touches when clenching a fist, as shown in Fig. 20) touching the two acupoints of Shenshu (1.5 cun away from the spinous process of the second lumbar vertebra). Rub the acupoints up and down 36 times. (See Fig. 59)

Turn the palms outward, clenching the fists slightly, the nails of the fingers not touching the palms. The acupoints of Outer Laogong (at the back of the hand opposite the Inner Laogong in the palms) should now touch the two acupoints of Shenshu. Stand this way for 20 minutes (as shown in Fig. 60).

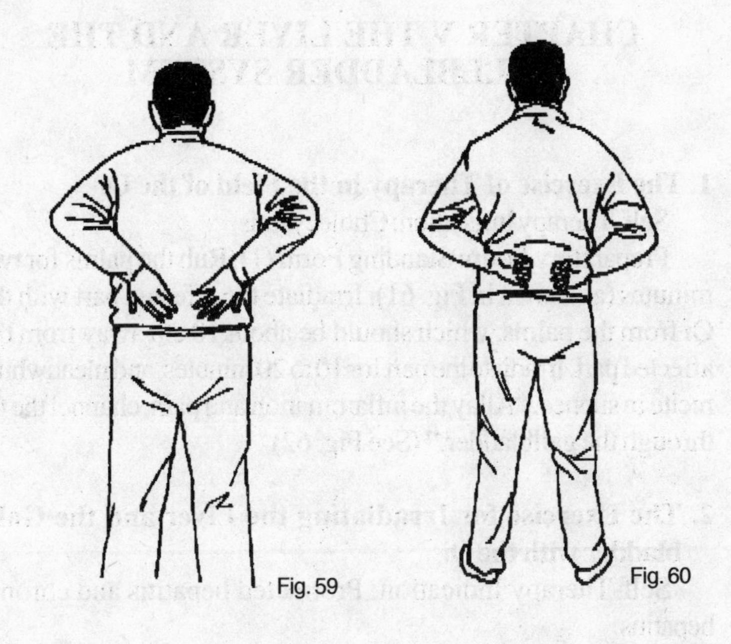

Fig. 59 Fig. 60

CHAPTER V THE LIVER AND THE GALLBLADDER SYSTEM

1. The Exercise of Therapy in the Field of the Qi

Self-Therapy Indication: Cholecystitis.

Preparatory Form: Standing Form (1). Rub the palms for two minutes (as shown in Fig. 61). Irradiate the affected part with the Qi from the palms, which should be about 10 cm away from the affected part. Irradiate the part for 10 to 20 minutes, and meanwhile, recite in silence, "Allay the inflammation and pain, channel the Qi through the gallbladder." (See Fig. 62)

2. The Exercise for Irradiating the Liver and the Gallbladder with the Qi

Self-Therapy Indication: Protracted hepatitis and chronic hepatitis.

Preparatory Form: Standing Form (2).

1) Relax the whole body. Stretch your arms out to the left and right. Make a circle forward and upward with the hands, the hands closing in front of the chest. Visualise the point where the two palms touch for 5 minutes (as shown in Fig. 63). Separate the hands, the palms facing in. Direct the left palm to the upper part of the right breast, keeping the palm 10 cm away from the breast. Direct the right palm to the lower part of the right breast at the same distance. Bend the knees slightly, imagining that two hot streams are flowing from the palms into the liver, green as in the liver being discharged through the acupoints of Yongquan (in the middle point of the sole of the foot, in the pit formed when the toes

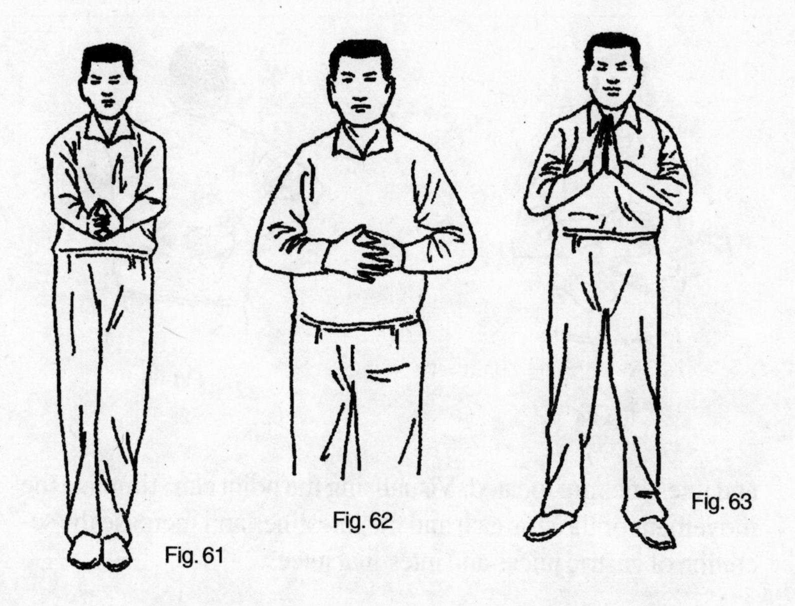
Fig. 61 Fig. 62 Fig. 63

bend, as shown in Fig. 25) to the ground. (See Fig. 64)

2) Rub the hands until they are warm. Keep the acupoints of Inner Laogong (above the transverse line, between the second and third metacarpal bones, where the middle finger tip touches when clenching a fist, as shown in Fig. 20) pressing the acupoins of Danshu (at both sides between the tenth and eleventh thoracic vertebrae at the back) for 5 minutes (as shown in Fig. 65).

3. The Exercise for Visualising the Acupoint of Dantian

Self-Therapy Indication: This can recover and strengthen the function of the liver, the pancreas, the gallbladder, the intestines and the stomach.

Preparatory Form: Standing Form (2). Relax the whole body, visualising the acupoint of Middle Dantian (which is in the pit of the stomach, as shown in Fig. 66). This point is where the pylorus

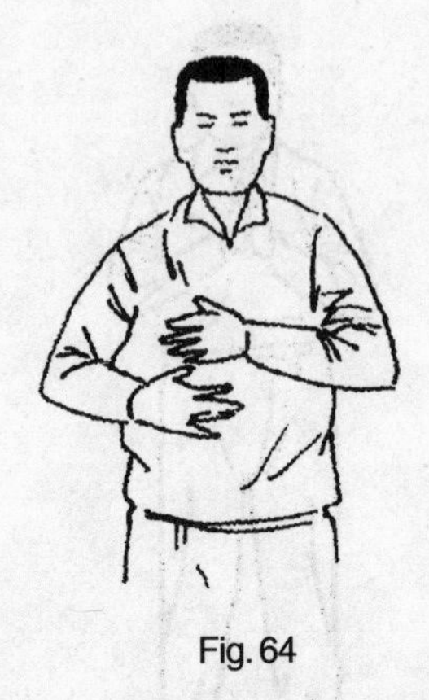
Fig. 64

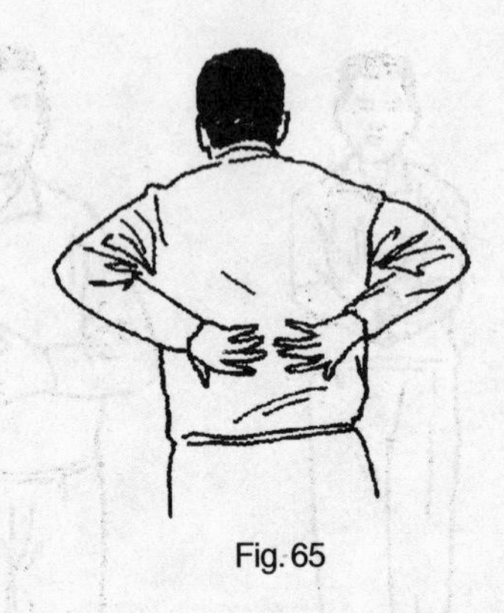
Fig. 65

and intestines are located. Visualising the point can stimulate the movement of the stomach and the intestines and increase the secretion of gastric juices and intestinal juices.

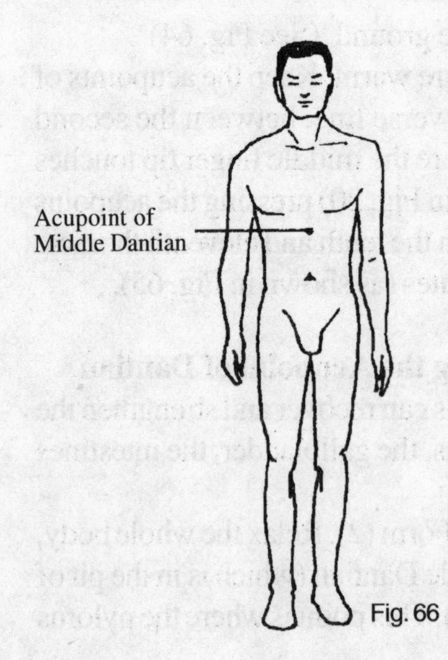

Fig. 66

4. The Exercise of Massaging the Acupoints of Zhangmen

Self-Therapy Indication: Cirrhosis of the liver.

Preparatory Form: Standing Form (2). Relax the whole body, rubbing the palms until they are warm. Massage the acupoints of Zhangmen (at both sides of the abdomen, below the free end of the eleventh floating rib). Massaging the acupoints up and down makes one cycle, which should be repeated 64 times. (See Fig. 67)

Then bend the knees and

squat at an angle of 60 degrees with the hands closed in front of the chest. After visualising the acupoints of Laogong (for the location, see Fig. 20) for 5 minutes, as shown in Fig. 68, separate the hands and direct the palms to the acupoints of Zhangmen, and the distance between the palm and the acupoint is about 10 cm. Irradiate the acupoints with the palms for 10 to 15 minutes. (See Fig. 69)

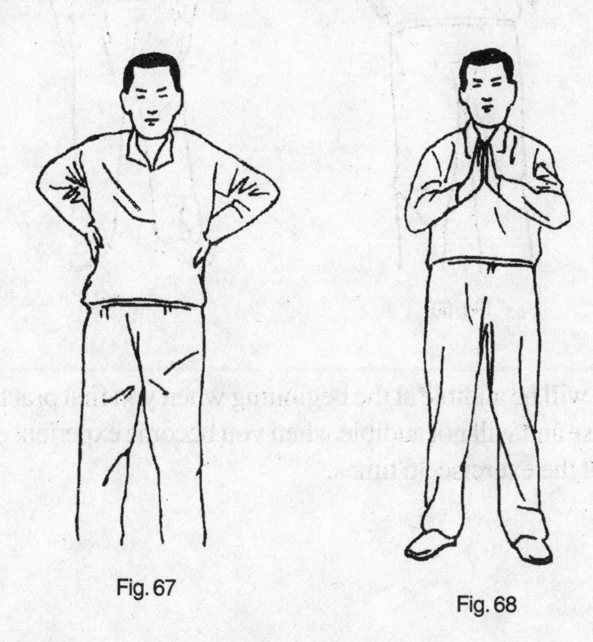

Fig. 67

Fig. 68

5. The Exercise for Producing Sound to Channel the Qi

Self-Therapy Indication: Diseases in the liver.

Preparatory Form: Standing Form (2). Relax the whole body and stand still for 5 minutes. Breathe through the abdomen by throwing the abdomen out when inhaling (as shown in Fig. 70) and pulling it in when exhaling. Inhale as deeply as possible and exhale thoroughly. Produce the sound of "her" when exhaling. The

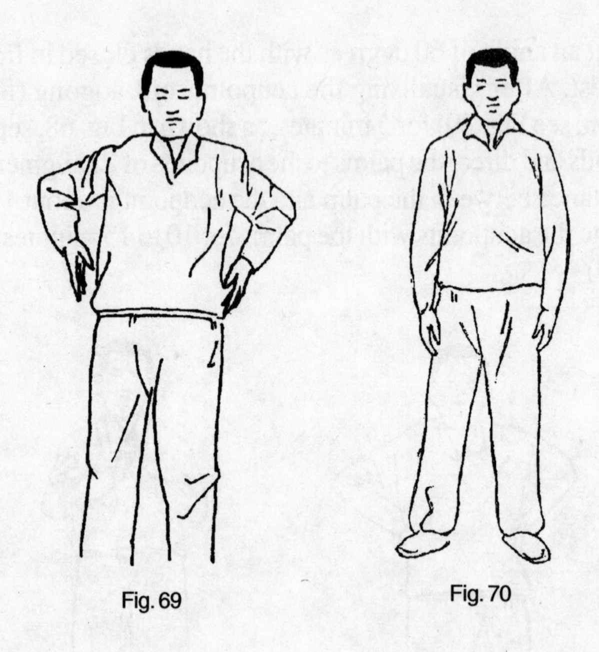

Fig. 69 Fig. 70

sound will be audible at the beginning when you first practise the exercise and will not audible when you become experienced at it. Repeat the exercise 36 times.

CHAPTER VI THE GASTROENTERIC SYSTEM

1. The Exercise of the Six-Circle Movement

Self-Therapy Indication: Chronic gastroenteritis, diabetes, arthritis and lumbago. The exercise has an effect of massaging the internal organs and strengthening the immunity of the organs.

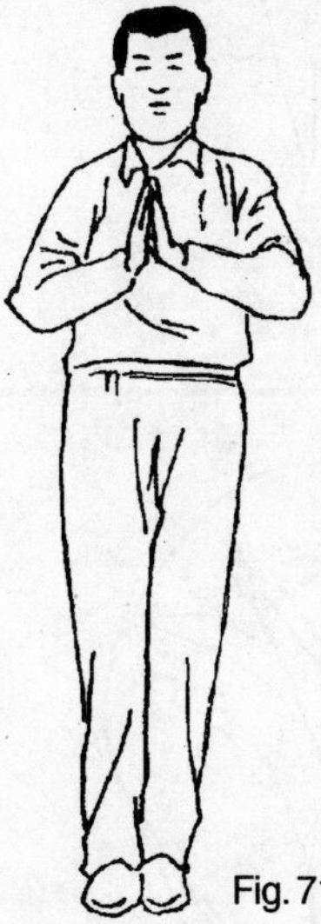

Fig. 71

Preparatory Form: Standing Form (1). Look forward. Realax the shoulders and elbows. Stretch the arms out to the left and right, then move the arms in circling motion until the hands are close and pointing upward in front of the chest. The acupoints of Laogong (for the location see Fig. 20) touch each other gently. Visualise the centre of the palms, as shown in Fig. 71.

Start the first circling movement, with hands moving to the left and then toward the upper-front and round the head. The eyes must always follow the hands. When the hands move to the left, turn the waist and the hip to the right. When the hands turn to the right, turn the waist and the hip to the left, with the movement of the hands always in the opposite direction to that of the waist and the hip (as shown in Fig. 72 and Fig. 73). After the first circling movement around the head, move the hands back to the front of the chest. Bend the knees slightly and start the second circling movement. Move the hands to the left and around the knees (as shown in Fig. 74 and Fig. 75).

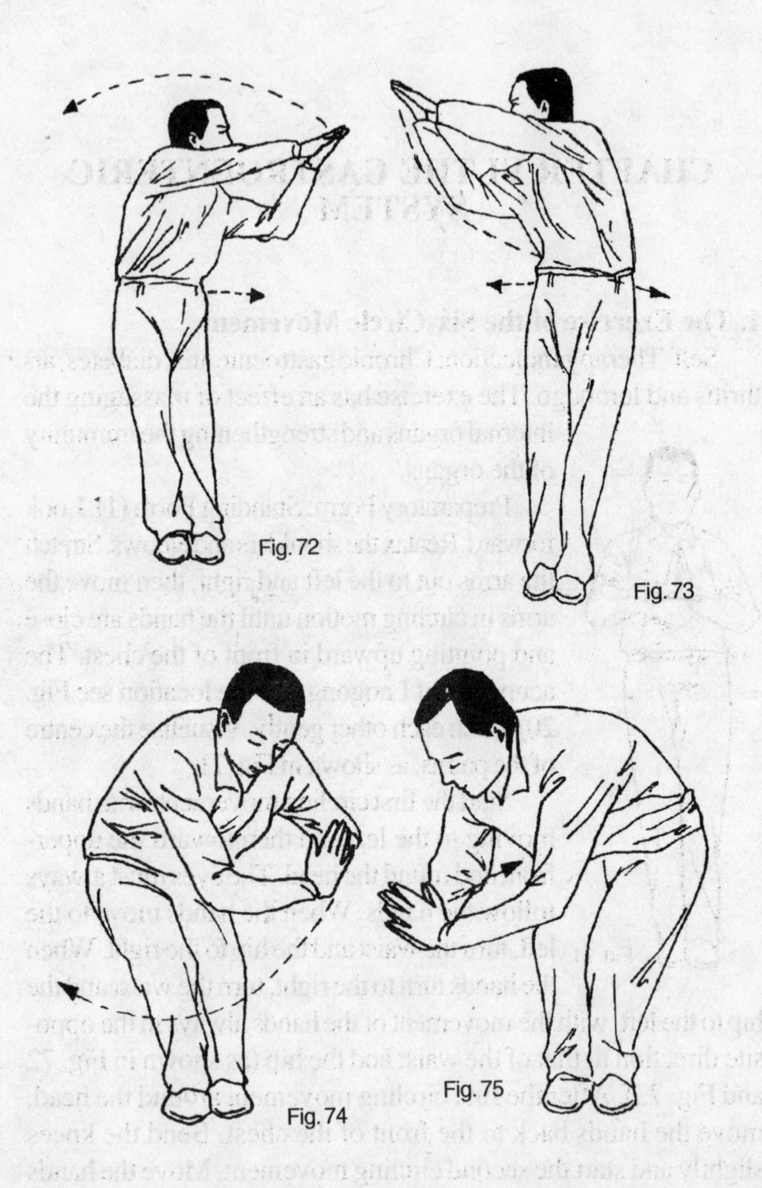

Fig. 72

Fig. 73

Fig. 74

Fig. 75

After the second circling movement around the knees, straighten the legs. Then start the third circling movement by moving the hands from the lower abdomen and around the chest. After circling, straighten the arms in front of the lower abdomen. (See Fig. 76, Fig. 77 and Fig. 78)

Turn the left palm up and bend the left elbow backward. Start the fourth circling movement by moving the hands to the left, above the left hip, with the right forearm pressing the left ribs (as shown in Fig. 79). After turning the thumbs up and turning the waist, move the hands back to the middle of the body. (See Fig. 80)

Turn the right palm up and bend the right elbow backward. Start the fifth circling movement by moving the hands to the right above the right hip, with the right forearm pressing the right ribs (as shown in Fig. 81). Then turn the thumbs up and turn the waist, moving the hands back to the front of the body, and stretching the arms forward. (See Fig. 82)

Raise the hands forward and upward over the head and then move downward (as shown in Fig. 83). Start the six circling movement. Stop the hands in front of the chest. (See Fig. 84)

Closing Form: Separate the little fingers first, and then the third, the middle, the forefingers and the thumbs, respectively. Relax the shoulders and the elbows, the hands hanging down naturally at the outside of the thighs (as shown in Fig. 85). Repeat the exercise 6 times.

2. The Exercise for Invigorating the Function of the Spleen and the Stomach

Self-Therapy Indication: Gastritis, gastric neuralgia and indigestion.

Preparatory Form: Standing Form (2). Relax the entire body. Move the left hand to the front of the chest, the palm facing inward and the tips of the fingers pointing to the right. Keep the acupoint of Hegu (a point in the middle of the hollow part between

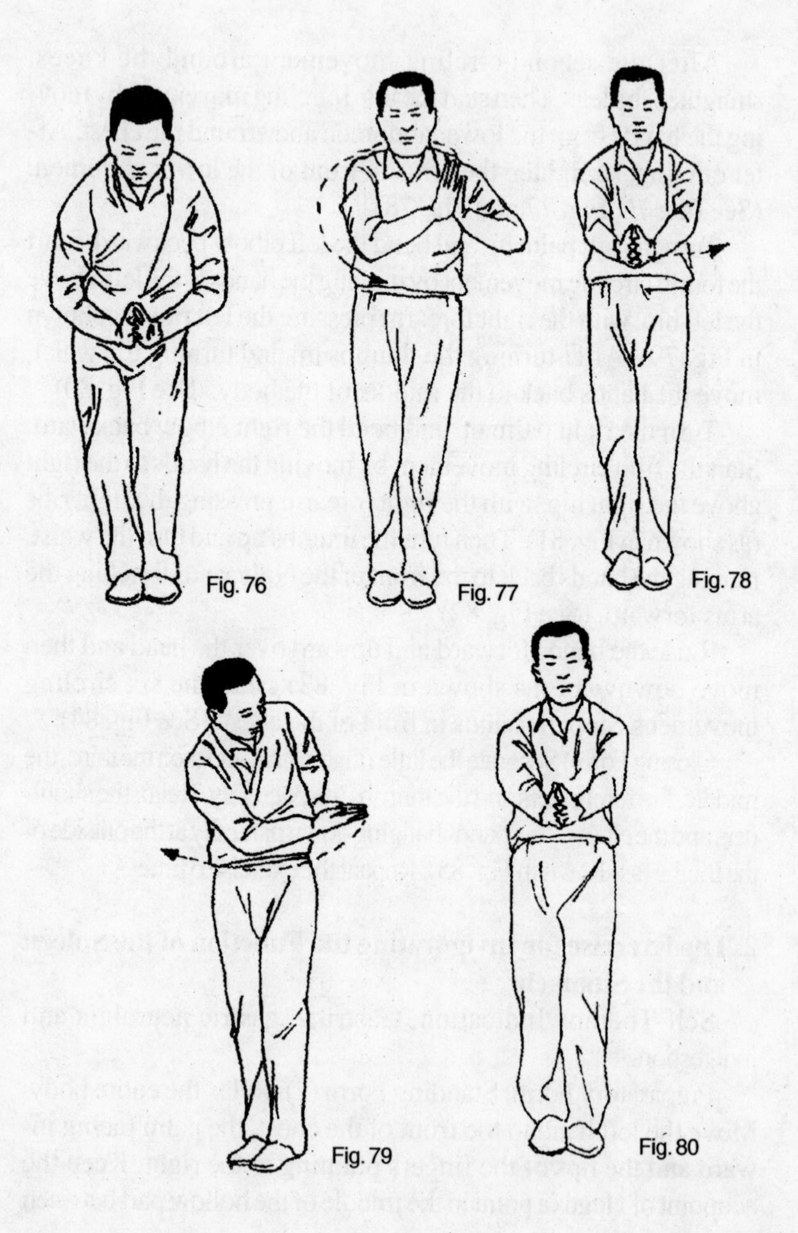

Fig. 76 Fig. 77 Fig. 78

Fig. 79 Fig. 80

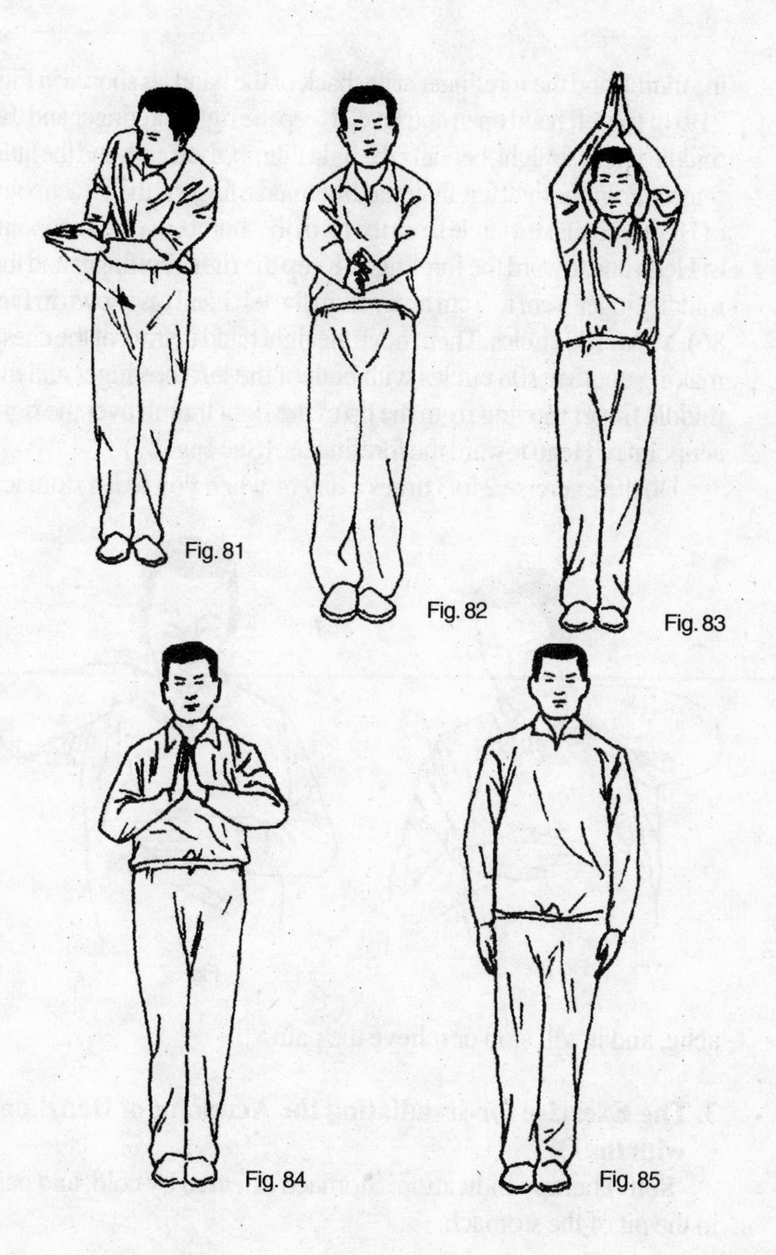

Fig. 81 Fig. 82 Fig. 83 Fig. 84 Fig. 85

the thumb and the forefinger at the back of the hand, as shown in Fig. 219) of the left hand open and level. Keep the right forefinger and the middle finger straight, bending the right thumb, the fourth and the little fingers. Point the right forefinger and the middle finger at the left acupoint of Hegu and make a circle from the tip of the thumb, over the acupoint of Hegu and toward the forefinger. Keep the right forefinger and the middle finger 3 cm to 5 cm away from the left hand (as shown in Fig. 86). Make 108 circles. Then move the right hand in front of the chest, making another 108 circles with both of the left forefinger and the middle finger moving from the tip of the right thumb over the right acupoint of Hegu toward the forefingers. (See Fig. 87)

Do the exercise 2 to 3 times a day or when you feel a stomach

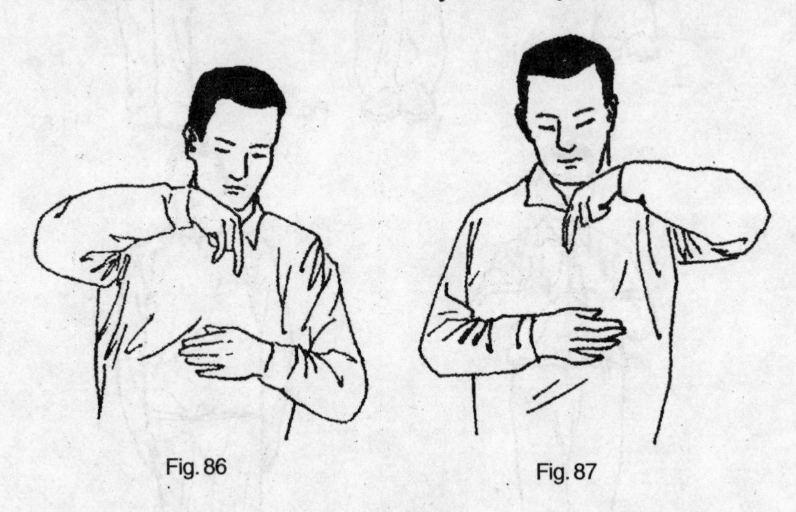

Fig. 86 Fig. 87

ache, and it will stop or relieve the pain.

3. The Exercise for Irradiating the Acupoint of Danzhong with the Qi

Self-Therapy Indication: Stomach affected by cold, and pain in the pit of the stomach.

Preparatory Form: Standing Form (3). Relax the whole body. Bend the knees slightly, with the hands closing in front of the chest (as shown in Fig. 88). Keep the eyes nearly closed, locking at the middle fingers for 5 minutes. If you are a man or boy, direct the left palm to the point 1.6 cm below the acupoint of Danzhong (in the middle line of the chest in a hollow between the breasts, as shown in Fig. 19), with the distance apart being 5 cm to 10 cm. Direct the right acupoint of Inner Laogong (above the transverse line, between the second and the third metacarpal bones, where the middle finger tip touches when clenching a fist, as shown in Fig. 20) to the left acupoint of Outer Laogong (at the back of the hand opposite the acupoint of Inner Laogong in the palm), the distance between the two hands being 5 cm to 10 cm. Stand for 10 to 20 minutes each session. If you are female, keep the right hand inside the left hand. Refer to the movement for males for further details about how to do the exercise if you are female. (See Fig. 89)

4. The Exercise of Moxibustion at the Acupoint of Shishang

Self-Therapy Indication: Distension of the abdomen, dypspepsia caused by excessive eating and the stomach affected by cold.

Sit on a chair or in an armchair. Administer moxibustion at the acupoints of Shishangmingjiu (beside the toes, at the joint of the second metatarsus, the distal portion of hallux, one in each sole, as shown in Fig. 90) with moxarolls for 20 minutes and administer this twice a day.

5. The Exercise of Massaging the Abdomen and the Feet

Self-Therapy Indication: Acid regurgitation and esophagospasm.

Preparatory Form: Standing Form (2). Relax the whole body.

Connect the two thumbs and two forefingers. Press the lower abdomen with the acupoints of Inner Laogong (above the transverse line, between the second and the third metacarpal bones, where the middle finger tip touches when clenching a fist, as shown in Fig. 20). Imagine there is a mass of hot air in the lower abdomen. Turn the mass of hot air clockwise with the hands 36 times, and turn it counter-clockwise another 36 times (as shown in Fig. 91). Rub the heels up and down and repeat the up and down rubbing of each foot 108 times. It is desirable to rub the feet until they are warm and distanding.

6. The Exercise of Irradiating the Stomach and Moving the Toes

Self-Therapy Indication: Indigestion.

Preparatory Form: Either the Sitting Form or Standing Form (2) will do. Rub your hands together until they are warm. Direct the palms to the stomach, the distance in between being 10 cm. Your 10 toes should grasp the ground at the same time. Do the exercise for 10 minutes each time (as shown in Fig. 92 and Fig. 93). It's desirable to do the exercise one hour after a meal.

7. The Exercise for Channelling the Qi Through the Acupoints of Danshu

Self-Therapy Indication: Bitter taste.

Preparatory Form: Standing Form (2). Relax the whole body, rubbing the hands together until they are warm. Rub the two acupoints of Danshu (1.5 cun below on both sides of the tenth thoracic vertebra) up and down. Repeat the up and down rubbing 64 times. (See Fig. 94)

Roll up the tongue. Don't spit saliva. If there is any, swallow it. Try to keep the tongue in the rolled up position.

8. The Exercise of Lying on the Back to Channel the Qi

Self-Therapy Indication: Arresting vomitting.

Lie on your back, with the whole body relaxed. Stretch the

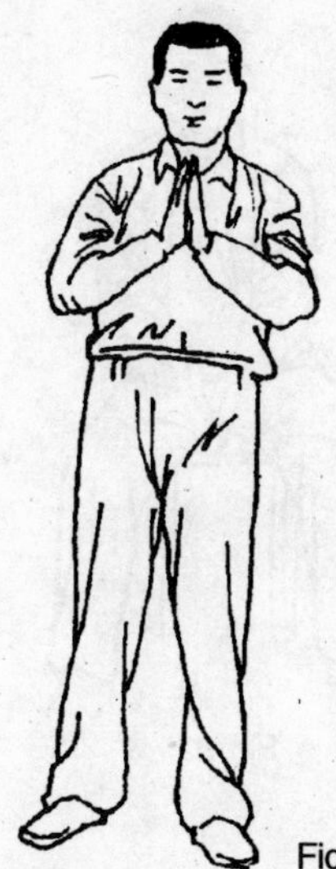

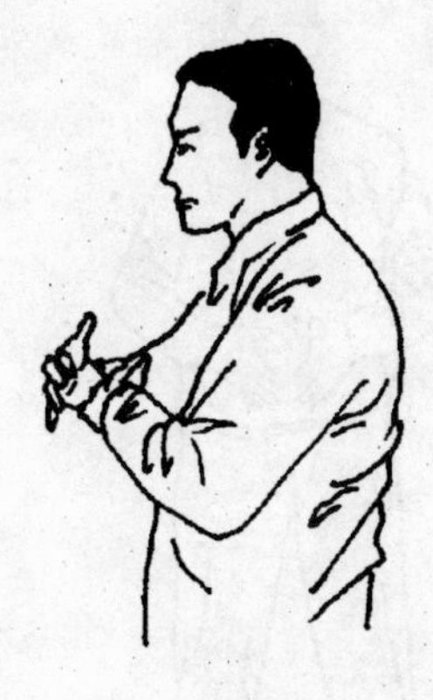

Fig. 89

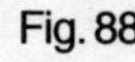

Fig. 88

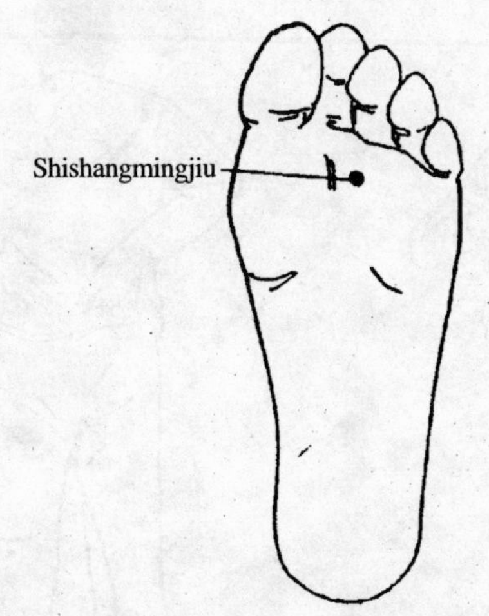

Fig. 90

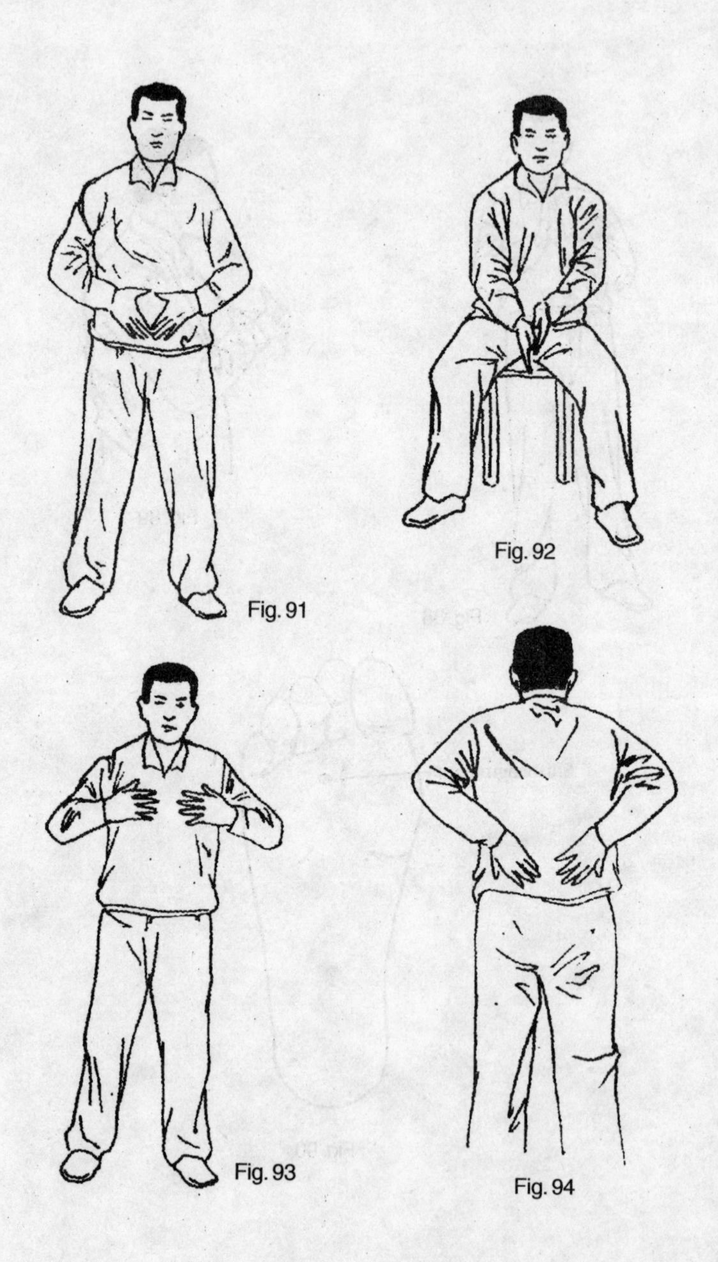

Fig. 91

Fig. 92

Fig. 93

Fig. 94

legs, putting the arms naturally at the two sides of the body (as shown in Fig. 95), and then put the left foot on top of the instep of the right foot. Breathe deeply and gently through the nasal passages 24 times (as shown in Fig. 96). Then put the right foot on top of the instep of the left foot. Breathe deeply and gently through the nasal passages another 24 times (as shown in Fig. 97).

9. The Exercise of Visualising the Fingers in Standing Form

Self-Therapy Indication: Vomit and diarrhea.

Preparatory Form: Standing Form (3). Relax the whole body. Raise the forearms to the angle of 10 degrees to the trunk. Keep the hands as high as the elbows and shoulder-width apart. Separate the ten fingers and relax them, visualising the central point of each nail. Imagine that the nails will come off the fingers. Stand this way for 10 to 20 minutes each time. (See Fig. 98)

10. The Exercise of Breathing While Bending the Neck Backwards to Channel the Qi

Self-Therapy Indication: Indigestion, dispelling the effects of alcohol.

Preparatory Form: Sitting Form. Relax the whole body. Bend the neck backward to face the sky. Inhale through the nasal passages and exhale through the mouth deeply and gently 24 times. (See Fig. 99).

11. The Exercise of Breathing to Channel the Qi

Self-Therapy Indication: The abdomen affected by cold, and stomach ache.

Lie on your back in a bed, with your feet shoulder-width apart, the toes pointing outward naturally. Relax the whole body (as shown in Fig. 100), breathing naturally 12 times. Then inhale deeply through the mouth and swallow the air before slowly exhaling it

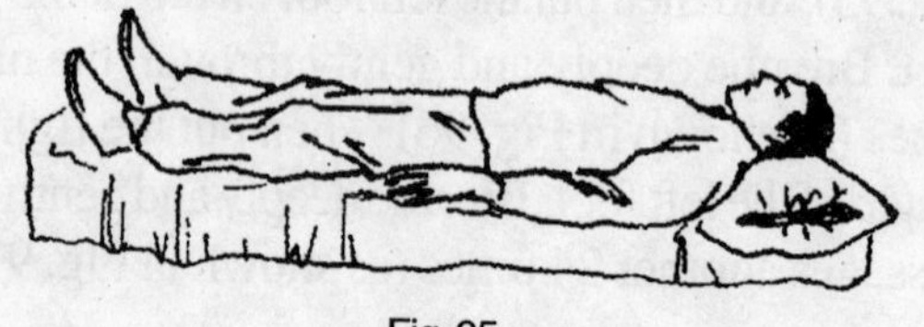

Fig. 95

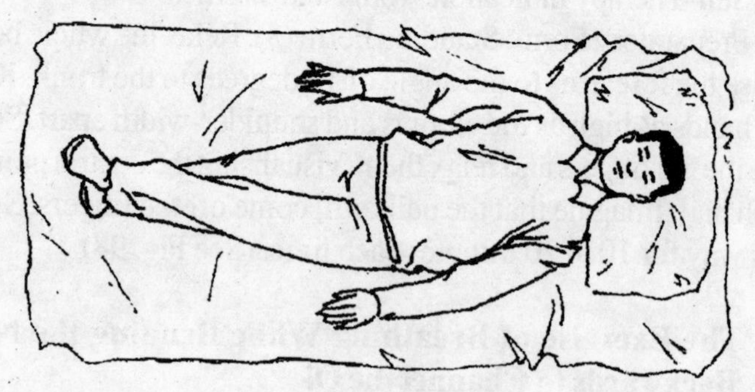

Fig. 96

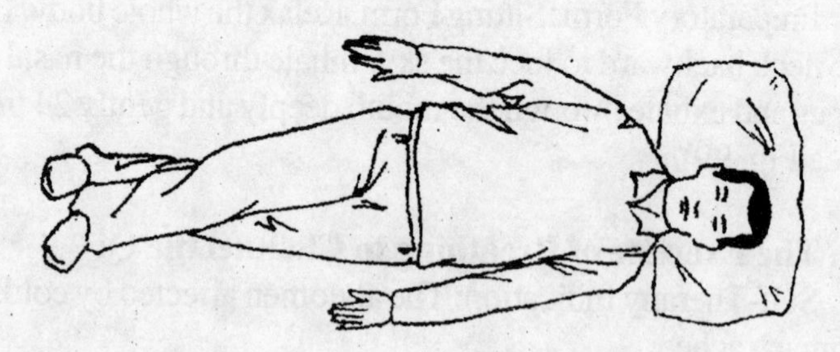

Fig. 97

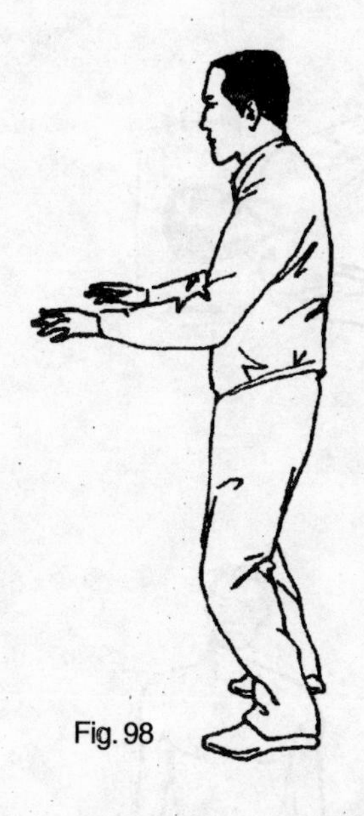
Fig. 98

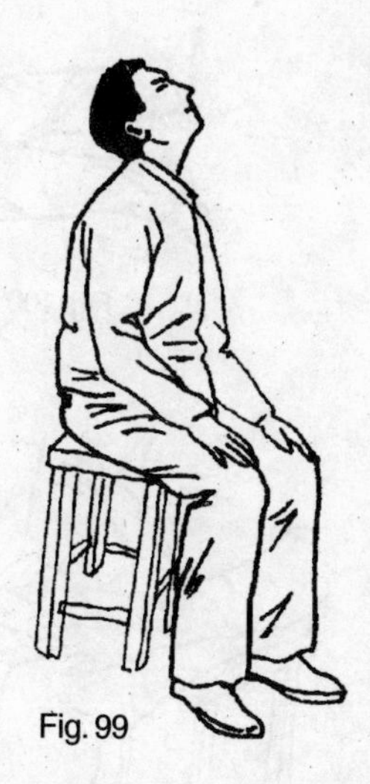
Fig. 99

out through the nasal passages. An inhalation and an exhalation make up one cycle, which should be repeated 36 times.

12. The Exercise of Rubbing the Feet to Conserve Health

Self-Therapy Indication: Distension of the abdomen and indigestion caused by improper diet or over-eating.

Sit on a chair or an armchair. Put the left foot on top of the right leg, rubbing hard the upper part of the left sole with the right palm. Repeat the up and down rubbing 108 times. Then put the right foot on the left leg and rub it with the left palm. Repeat the up and down rubbing another 108 times. (See Fig. 101)

13. The Exercise of Moxibustion at the Point Below the Navel

Self-Therapy Indication: Ascites and ringing in of the intestines.

Sit in an armchair or lie on a bed. Administer moxibustion at the point 1 cm below the navel for 15 minutes each time. (See Fig. 102)

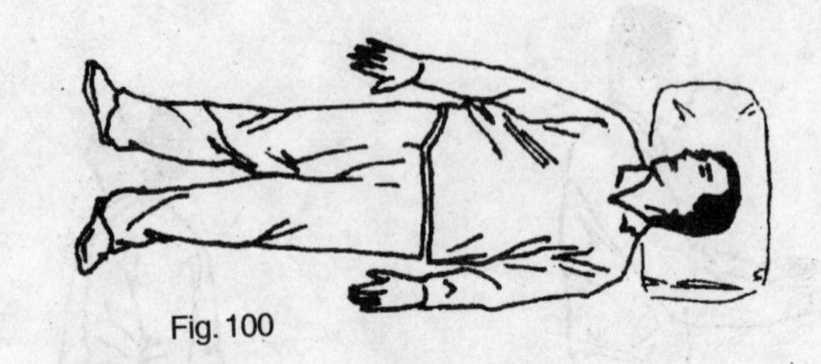

Fig. 100

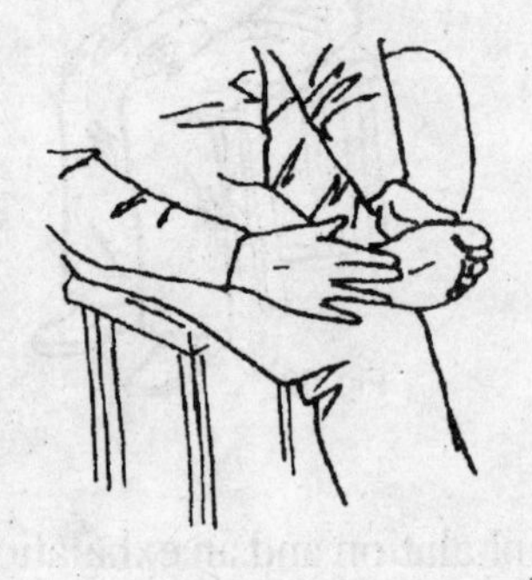

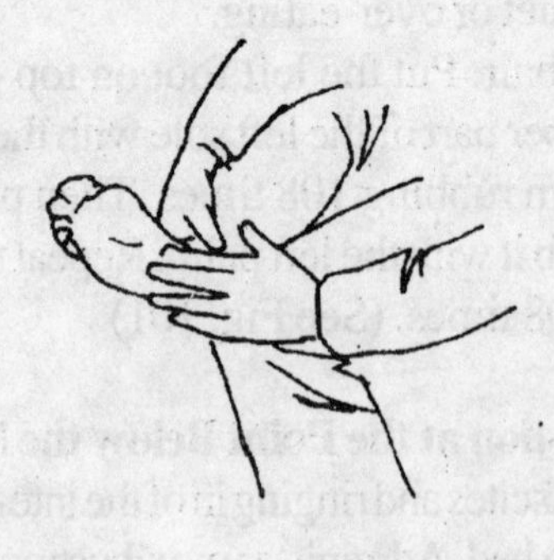

Fig. 101

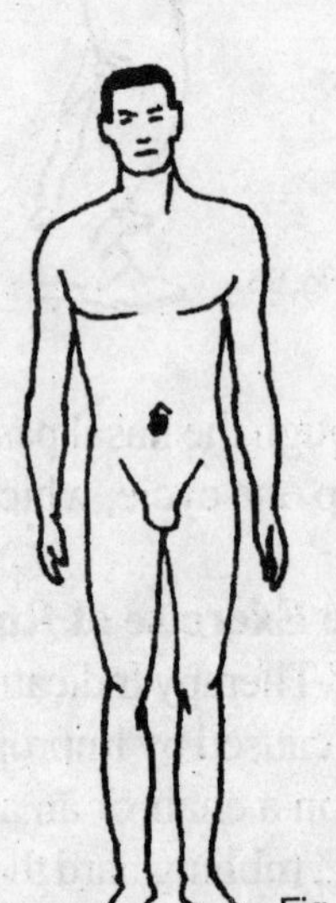

Fig. 102

14. The Exercise of Visualising the Acupoint of Zhangmen

Self-Therapy Indication: Diarrhea, indigestion, lumbago and backache.

Preparatory Form: Standing Form (2). Relax the whole body, visualising the acupoints of Zhangmen at the two sides of the abdomen, below the free ends of the eleventh floating ribs. Visualise the acupoints for 20 minutes each time and twice a day, once in the morning and once in the evening. (See Fig. 103)

15. The Exercise of Visualising the Acupoint of Qihai

Self-Therapy Indication: Diseases in the large and small intestines, and the urinary bladder.

Preparatory Form: Standing Form (2). Relax the whole body. Visualise the acupoint of Qihai 1.5 cun below the navel. Visualise the acupoint for 20 minutes. Do the exercise every morning and evening. (See Fig. 104)

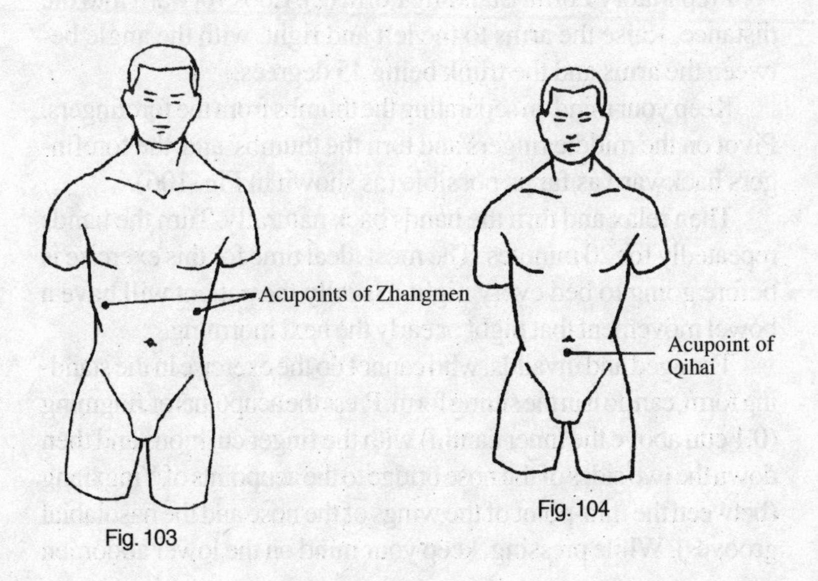

Fig. 103

Fig. 104

16. The Exercise for Inhibiting Over-Frequent Urination

Self-Therapy Indication: Chronic enteritis, chronic dysentery, and over-frequent urination.

Preparatory Form: Standing Form (2). Look forward into the distance. Raise the arms to the left and right, the angle between the arms and the trunk being 45 degrees. Keep the palms facing forward, the thumbs pointing up and the acupoints of Hegu (as shown in Fig. 219) open. Concentrate your mind on the thumbs and the forefingers. Turn the thumbs forward and downward as far as possible. Then relax the fingers and turn them back to the former position. Repeat the turning for 20 minutes. It is better to do the exercise every morning and evening. (See Fig. 105)

17. The Exercise for Curing Constipation

Self-Therapy Indication: Gerontological constipation and habitual constipation.

Preparatory Form: Standing Form (2). Look forward into the distance. Raise the arms to the left and right, with the angle between the arms and the trunk being 45 degrees.

Keep your mind on separating the thumbs from the forefingers. Pivot on the middle fingers and turn the thumbs and the forefingers backward as far as possible (as shown in Fig. 106).

Then relax and turn the hands back naturally. Turn the hands repeatedly for 20 minutes. The most ideal time for this exercise is before going to bed every night. Usually the patient will have a bowel movement that night or early the next morming.

The aged and invalids, who cannot do the exercise in the standing form, can do it in the sitting form. Press the acupoints of Jingming (0.1 cun above the inner canthi) with the finger cushions and then down the two sides of the nose bridge to the acupoints of Yingxiang (between the min-point of the wings of the nose and the nasolabial grooves). While pressing, keep your mind on the lower abdomen and the anus. Repeat these movements 108 times. Do the exercise every morning and evening.

18. The Exercise of Rubbing the Ribs to Channel the Qi

Self-Therapy Indication: Constipation, and abdominal distension.

Lie on your back on a hard bed. Relax the whole body, freeing your mind from any thoughts. Rub, massage and press your ribs at the two sides in the front from the breasts down to the lower abdomen (as shown in Fig. 107) and in the back from the armpits downwards for 5 to 10 minutes (as shown in Fig. 108).

Then inhale through the mouth deeply and swallow the air before you exhale through the nasal passages. An inhalation and an exhalation make up one cycle, which should be repeated 36 times.

19. The Exercise of Breathing Like a Tortoise While Lying on the Back

Self-Therapy Indication: Constipation, and not having a bowel movement for days.

Lie on your back on a bed, relaxing the whole body. Cover the body with a quilt, with your head uncovered and holding the upper side of the quilt with your hands. (As shown in Fig. 109). Imagine that there is air in the lower abdomen, making 36 counter clockwise rotations and then make 36 anticlockwise rotations. After that, inhale deeply and swallow the air, and shrink your head under the quilt as far as possible (as shown in Fig. 110) before sticking your head out of the quilt and exhaling slowly. Breathe 24 times in this way.

20. The Exercise of Moving the Toes to Channel the Qi

Self-Therapy Indication: Eructation and a lump in the abdomen.

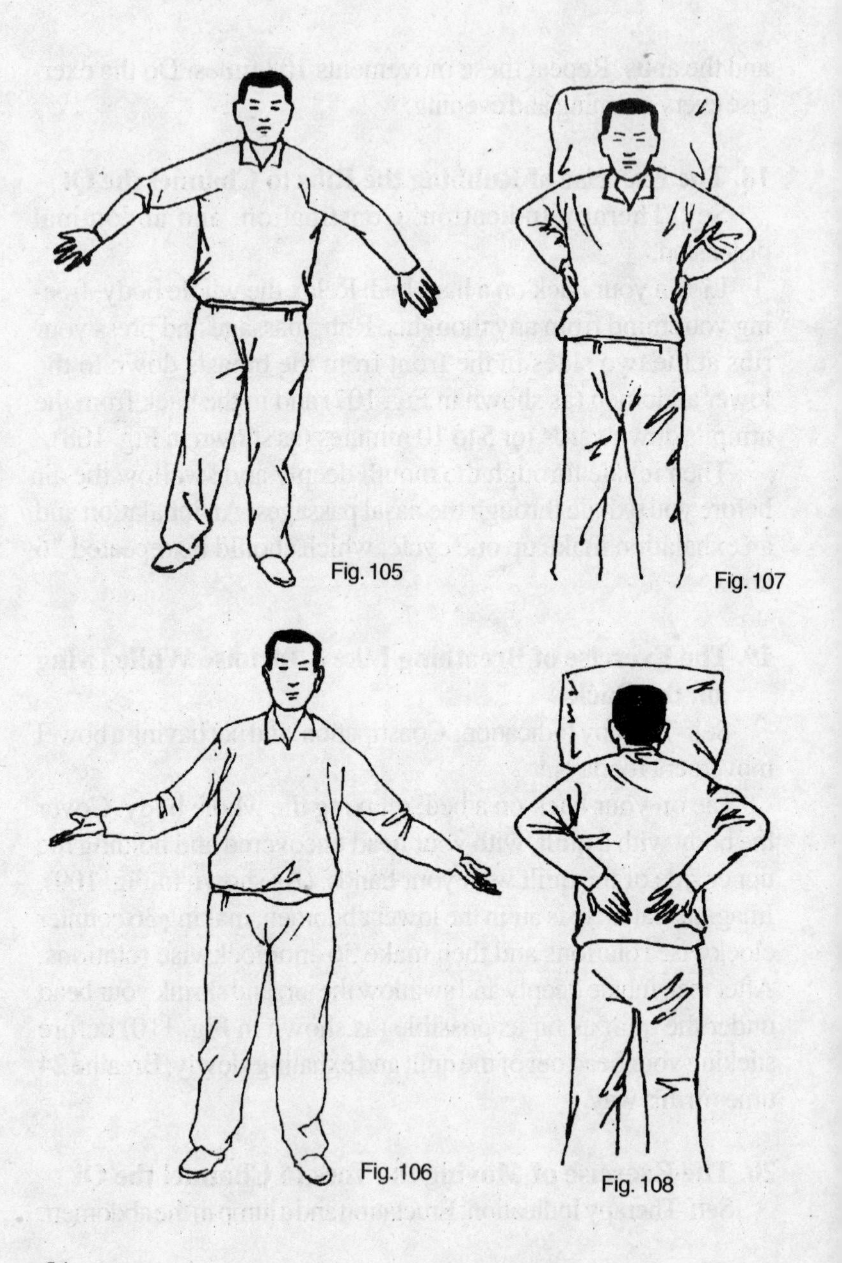

Fig. 105 Fig. 107

Fig. 106 Fig. 108

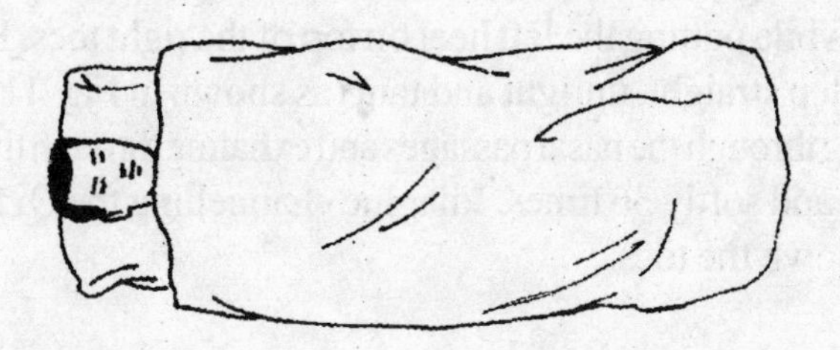

Fig. 109

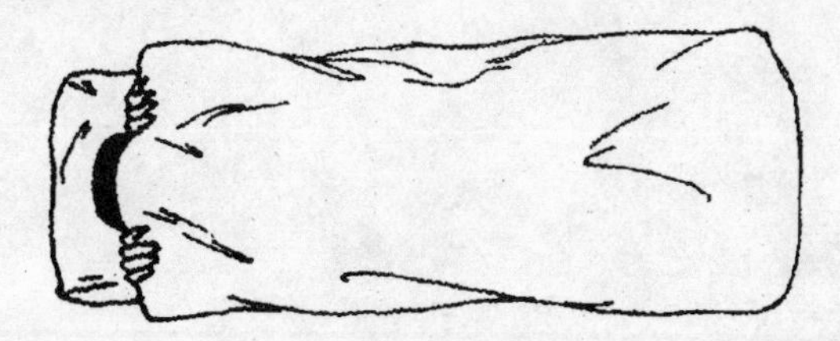

Fig. 110

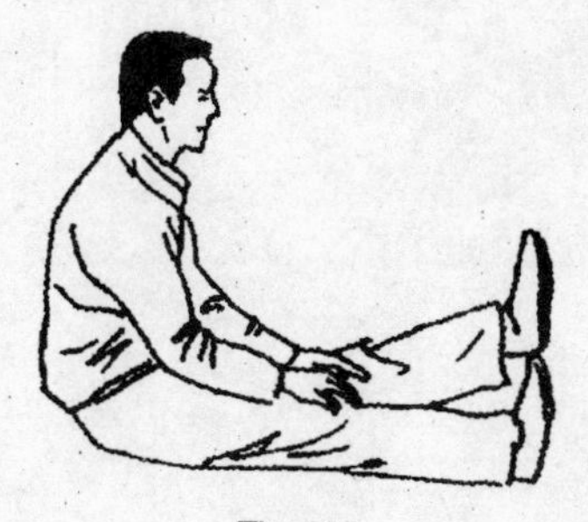

Fig. 111

Sit straight up on a hard bed. Relax the whole body, straightening the legs, and keeping the toes of the right foot upward and stable while putting the left heel on top of the right toes. Keep the left instep straight, upright and taut (as shown in Fig. 111) while inhaling through the nasal passages and exhaling through the mouth deeply and softly 36 times. Imagine channelling the Qi from the chest down the toes.

CHAPTER VII THE RESPIRATORY SYSTEM

1. The Exercise of Holding the Breath to Channel the Qi

Self-Therapy Indication: Cough and eructation.

Preparatory From: Standing Form (2). Relax the whole body.

Inhale deeply and gently through the nasal passages while turning the head slowly to the left. (As shown in Fig. 112). Hold the breath for a while and then look forward before exhaling slowly. Then inhale deeply and gently through the nasal passages while turning the trunk backward (as shown in Fig. 113). Hold the breath for a while and then look backward before exhaling slowly. Return to the former position before repeating the movement mentioned above in the opposite direction (as shown in Fig. 114 and Fig. 115). Repeat the left-turning and the right-turning 6 times, respectively.

2. The Exercise of Exhaling by Coughing to Channel the Qi

Self-Therapy Indication: Cough and eructation.

Preparatory Form: Sitting Form. Relax the whole body (as shown in Fig. 116). Inhale deeply and gently through the nasal passages before holding the breath for a while. Cough so as to make the air flow upward from the chest and rush out through the throat. Exhale after coughing. Repeat the movements 12 or 24 times. Do the exercise once in every morning and evening.

3. The Exercise of Regulating the Breath to Induce Perspiration

Self-Therapy Indication: Cold.

Preparatory Form: Sitting Form. Relax the whole body (as shown in Fig. 117), freeing the mind from any thoughts and clos-

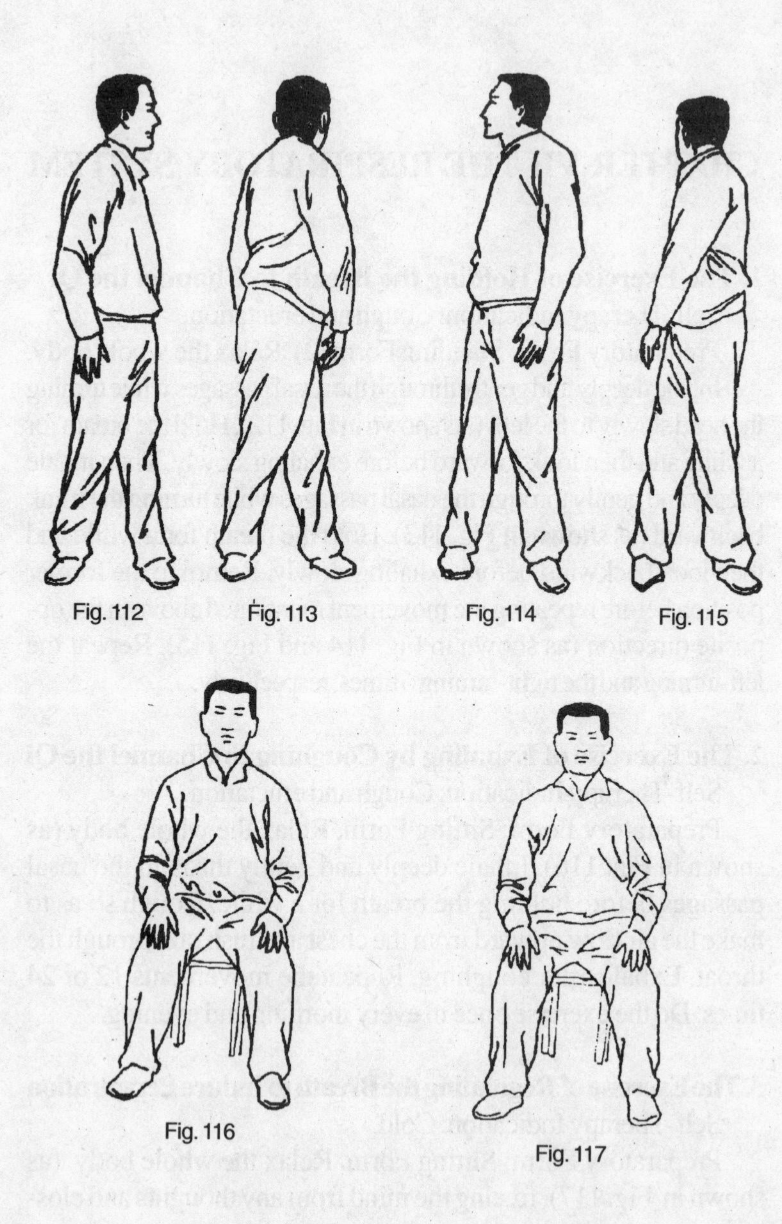

Fig. 112 Fig. 113 Fig. 114 Fig. 115

Fig. 116 Fig. 117

ing the eyes gently. Inhale deeply and gently through the nasal passages and hold the breath as long as possible after full inhalation. Then breathe the air out slowly. Do this kind of breathing until you perspire.

4. The Exercise of Massaging a Dry Rubdown

Self-Therapy Indication: Preventing influenza.

Both standing or sitting forms will do. Relax the whole body.

Rub the hands until they are warm (as shown in Fig. 118). Massage the face 36 times with your warm hands (as shown in Fig. 119). Then comb your hair with your fingers from the front to the back and to the side 64 times (as shown in Fig. 120), until you feel hot on the scalp. Then rub each sole of your feet with your hands 64 times (as shown in Fig. 121). Finally rub the chest, the abdomen and the lower back until you feel hot.

5. The Exercise of Pressing the Palms

Self-Therapy Indication: Pertussis.

Preparatory Form: Standing Form (2). Relax the whole body. Hold out your left hand forward and upward, with the palm facing up.

Press repeatedly the centre of the left palm 64 times with the right thumb before putting the left hand down. Hold out the right hand forward and upward, with the palm facing up. Repeatedly press the centre of the right palm 64 times with the left thumb. (See Fig. 122 and Fig. 123).

6. The Exercise of Regulating the Breath to Allay Fever

Self-Therapy Indication: Fever and backache.

Lie on the stomach with no pillow. Stretch the legs, with the feet close together. Put the arms by the sides of the body, and keep the mouth nearly closed. Breathe deeply and gently through the nasal passages. An inhalation and an exhalation make up one

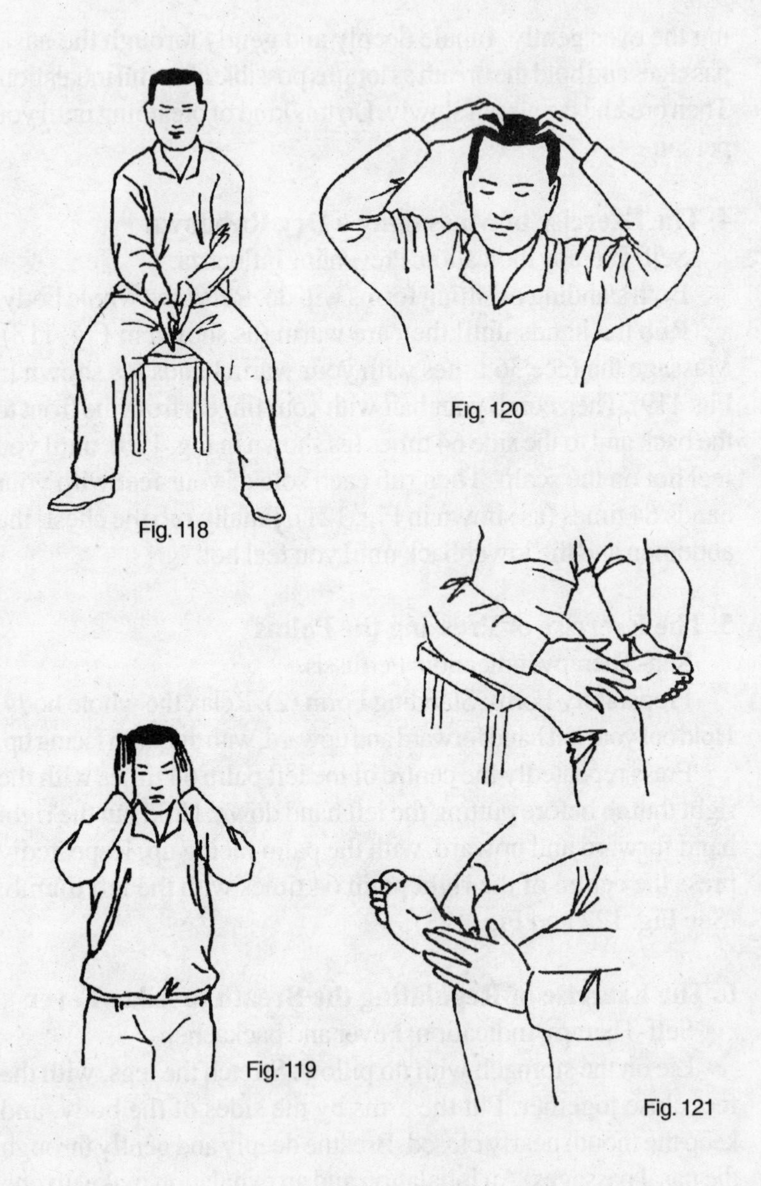

Fig. 118

Fig. 119

Fig. 120

Fig. 121

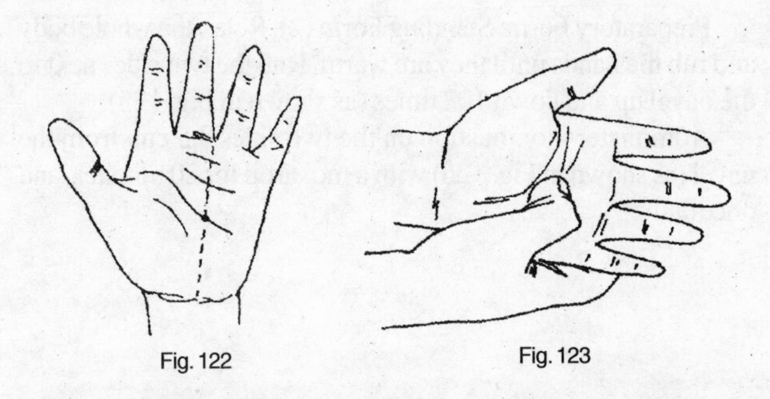

Fig. 122 Fig. 123

cycle. Repeat the cycle 64 times. Visualise the inhaled air as flowing into the lower abdomen when inhaling and flowing out through the sweat glands when exhaling. (See Fig. 124)

7. The Exercise of Rubbing and Moxibustion on the Abdomen

Self-Therapy Indication: Profuse sweating.

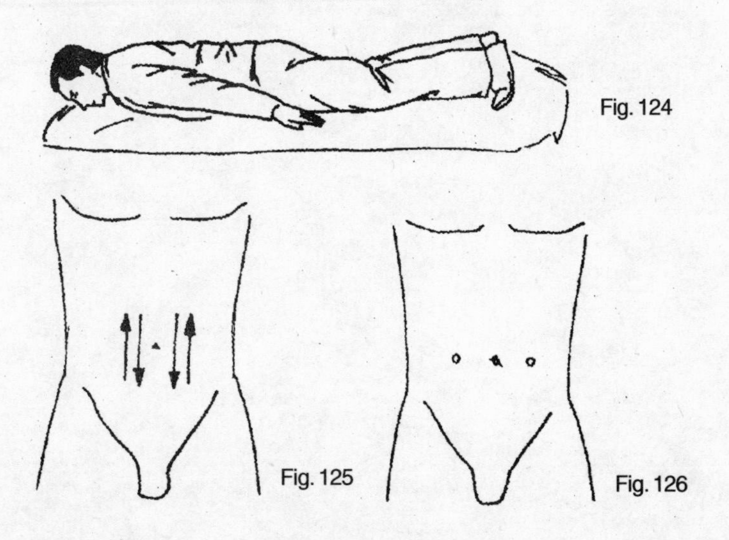

Fig. 124

Fig. 125 Fig. 126

Preparatory Form: Standing Form (2). Relax the whole body and rub the hands until they are warm. Rub the two sides next to the navel up and down 108 times (as shown in Fig. 125).

Administer moxibustion on the two sides 3.5 cun from the navel (as shown in Fig. 126) with a moxaroll for 20 minutes, and once daily.

CHAPTER VIII THE CENTRAL AND PERIPHERICAL NERVOUS SYSTEM

1. The Exercise of Moving the Vertebra

Self-Therapy Indication: This exercise can strengthen the function of the spinal nerves. It has a specially good effect on cervical vertebra diseases and psoatic strain.

Preparatory Form: Standing Form (2). Look straight ahead, moving the hands to the front of the thighs. Draw in the chest and the abdomen, bending the knees slightly, with hips lowered.

Lower the head slightly until the hands reach the knees (as shown in Fig. 127). Straighten the trunk slowly, thrust the chest out and bend the neck and spine backward (as shown in Fig. 128). Repeat the exercise 36 times.

2. The Exercise of Massaging the Acupoints of Xinshe

Self-Therapy Indication: Convulsion of the annuent muscle and an obstacle to the arm's movement.

Preparatory Form: Sitting Form. Sit upright, lowering the head slightly and relaxing the neck. Massage the two acupoints of Xinshe on each side of the neck (at the end of the transverse process of the fourth cervical vertebra outside the trapezius muscle, 1.5 cun below the back hairline, as shown in Fig. 129) 108 times. Do the exercise every morning and evening.

3. The Exercise of Turning the Arms to Regulate the Breath

Self-Therapy Indication: Pain and numbness in the arms.

Preparatory Form: Standing Form (1). Stand facing the south

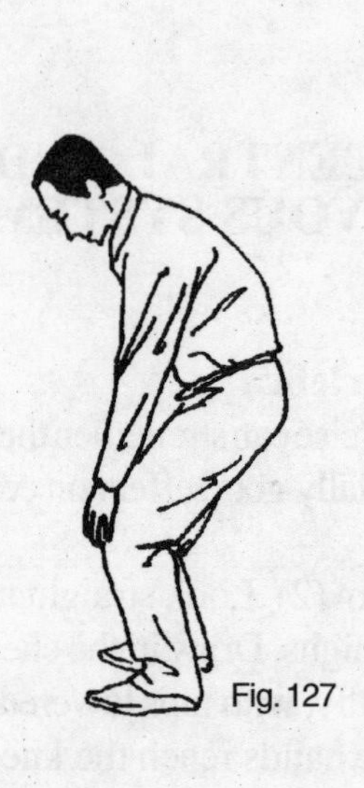

Fig. 127

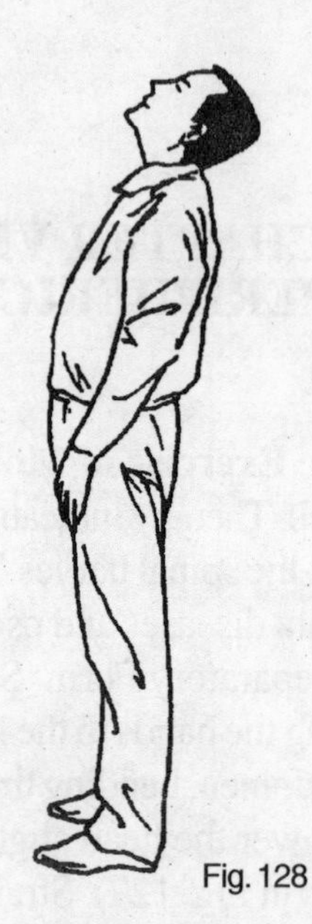

Fig. 128

and keep the body relaxed, freeing your mind from any thoughts (as shown in 130). Inhale slowly through the nasal passages, and imagine inhaling the air to the acupoint of Mingmen (in the hollow point below the spinous process of the second lumber vertebra, as shown in Fig. 57) before exhaling slowly while imagining that the air is flowing from the acupoint of Mingmen to the navel. Breathe in this way 36 times. Then look into the distance before stretching the arms forward and over the head, the palms facing each other and fingers pointing upward (as shown in Fig. 131). Turn the hands forward and outward 3 times (as shown in Fig. 132) and then backward and outward 3 times. Lower the hands down naturally. Repeat the movements mentioned above 7 times. Then lower the hands naturally by the sides of the body, turning the palms backwards and pushing back 7 times. While pushing slowly, imagine the pathogenic Qi is being discharged from the acupoints of

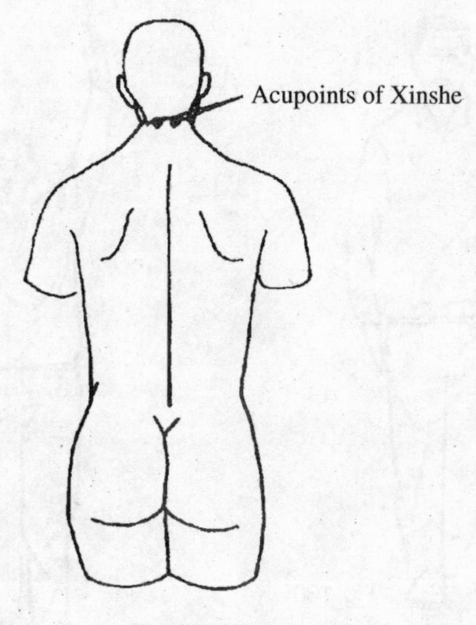

Fig. 129

Laogong (above the transverse line, between the second and the third metacarpal bones, where the middle finger tip touches when clenching a fist, as shown in Fig. 20). (See Fig. 133)

4. The Exercise of Visualising the Acupoints of Jianjing

Self-Therapy Indication: Omalaia, pain in the shoulder joints and multiplication in the shoulder joints.

Preparatory Form: Standing Form (2). Relax the whole body. Visualise the two acupoints of Jianjing (a point between the spinous process of the seventh cervical vertebra and the top of the shoulder, as shown in Fig. 134) for 20 minutes. This can strengthen the effect of the Qi and blood on the upper limbs and the physiological function of the arms. Do this exercise once overy morning and evening.

5. The Exercise for Relaxing the Shoulders, Elbows and Wrists

Self-Therapy Indication: Frozen shoulders; arthritis in the

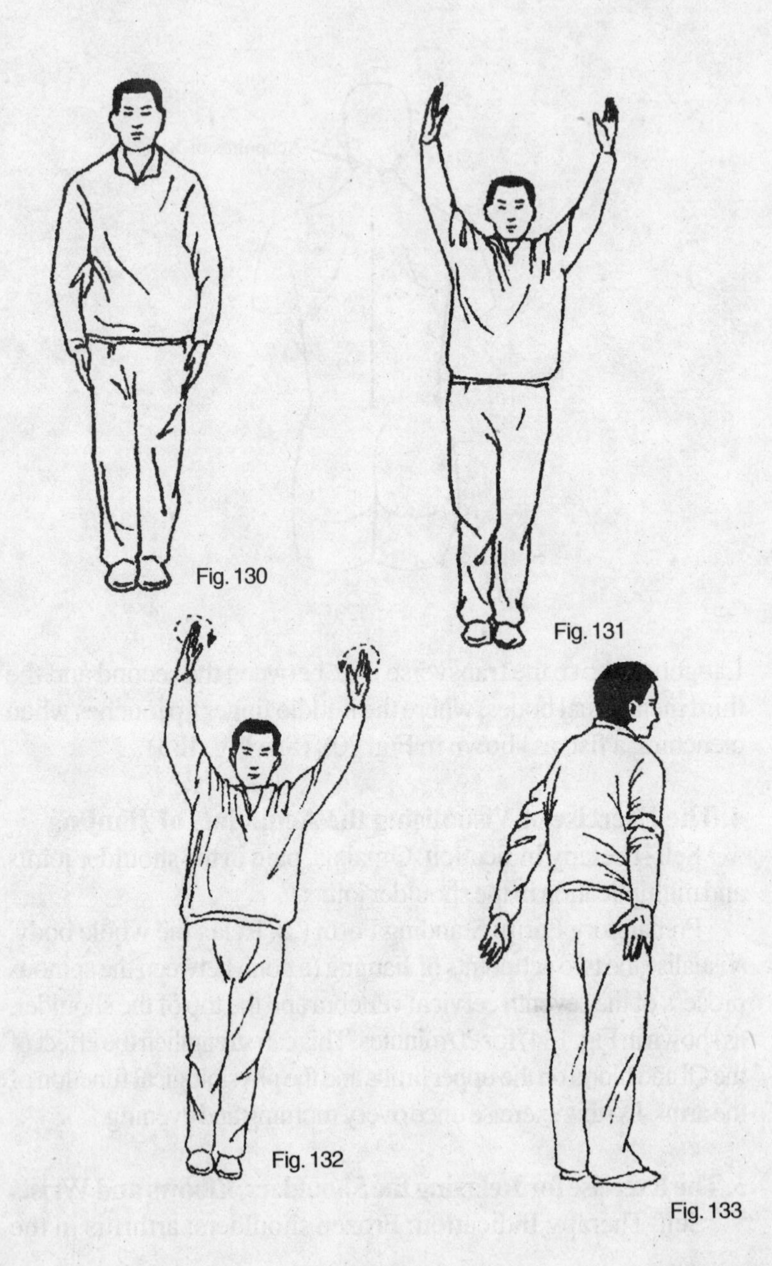

Fig. 130

Fig. 131

Fig. 132

Fig. 133

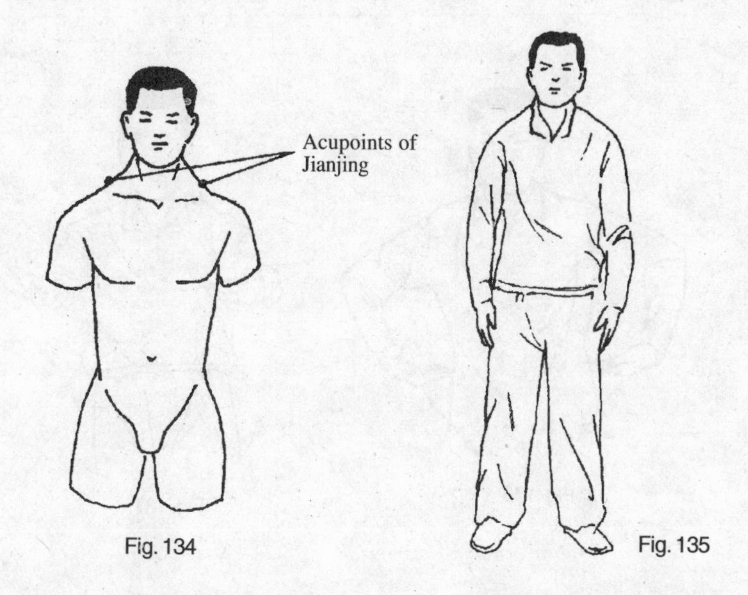

Fig. 134

Fig. 135

shoulders, elbows and wrists.

Preparatory Form: Standing Form (1). Look forward and relax the whole body (as shown in Fig. 135).

1) Raise both elbows upward, the palms facing up, the finger tips pointing at the ribs (as shown in Fig. 136). Then move the hands forward, straightening the arms so that they are shoulder-width apart and a little higher than the navel, the palms facing up and the finger nails pointing forward (as shown in Fig. 137).

2) Pivot the two palms, turning the hands outward and backward and connecting the middle fingers in front of the chest, while raising the hands to nose-height, the palms facing out and the thumbs pointing downward. (See Fig. 138)

3) Stretch the arms forward, with the backs of the hands touching each other, keep the hands straight at the shoulder-height and the thumbs pointing downward. (See Fig. 139).

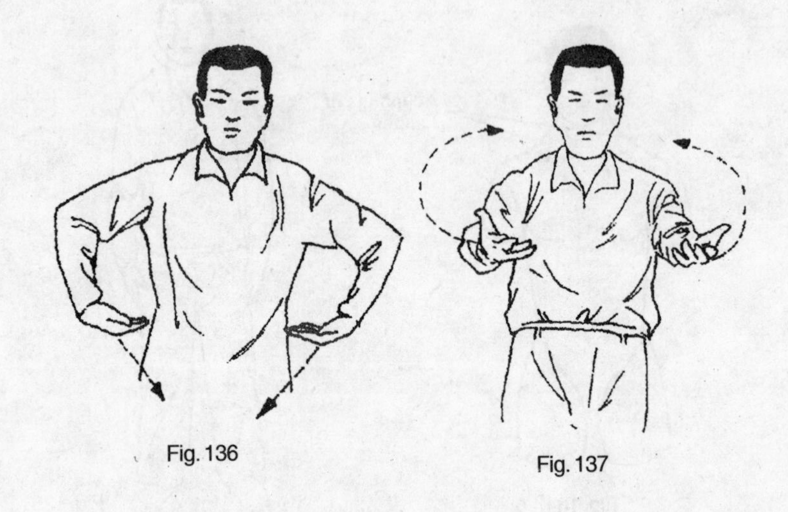

Fig. 136 Fig. 137

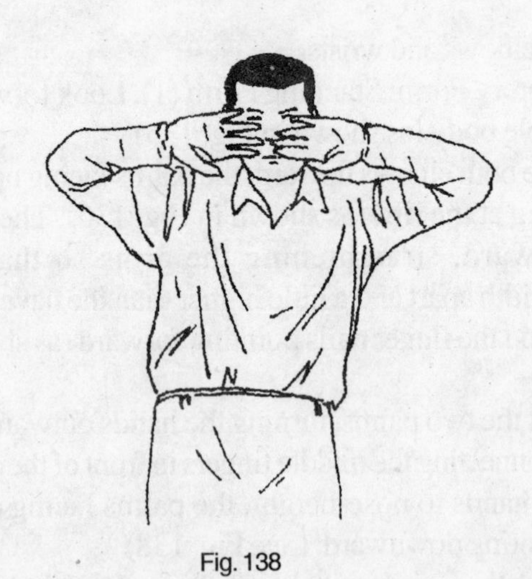

Fig. 138

4) Move the hands backward in an arc as if swimming. Connect the two hands at the acupoint of Mingmen (in a hollow below the spinous process of the second lumbar verterbra, as shown in Fig. 57), and connect the two acupoints of Hegu (whose locations are shown in Fig. 219), the palms facing up (as shown in Fig. 140).

5) Move the hands forward in an arc from the back to the front of the body, with the backs of the hands facing forward and touching each other, and the thumbs pointing down (as shown in Fig. 141).

6) Bend the elbows, keeping the hands in front of the chest, connecting the middle fingers, the palms facing forward and the thumbs pointing down. (See Fig. 142)

7) Turn the hands backward and outward and move the hands forward in an arc until the arms a little higher than the navel and at shoulder-width distance apart (as shown in Fig. 143).

8) Turn the hands inward and backward, and move them in an arc around the ribs to the acupoint of Mingmen at the back, connecting the acupoints of Hegu, with the palms facing up (as shown in Fig. 144). Drop the hands down naturally at the sides of the body. (See Fig. 145)

Repeat the eight-set movements 6 times.

6. The Exercise of Raising the Arms to Regulate the Breath

Self-Therapy Indication: Pain in the arms and shoulders, flaccidity of extremities.

Preparatory Form: Sitting Form. Relax the whole body, freeing your mind from any thoughts and breathing naturally through the nasal passages for 24 breaths (as shown in Fig. 146). Raise the left arm forward and upward, the palm facing up and the fingers pointing to the right (as shown in Fig. 147). Then raise the right arm and place the right hand, palm down, on top of the upturned left hand (as shown in Fig. 148). Breathe deeply and gently

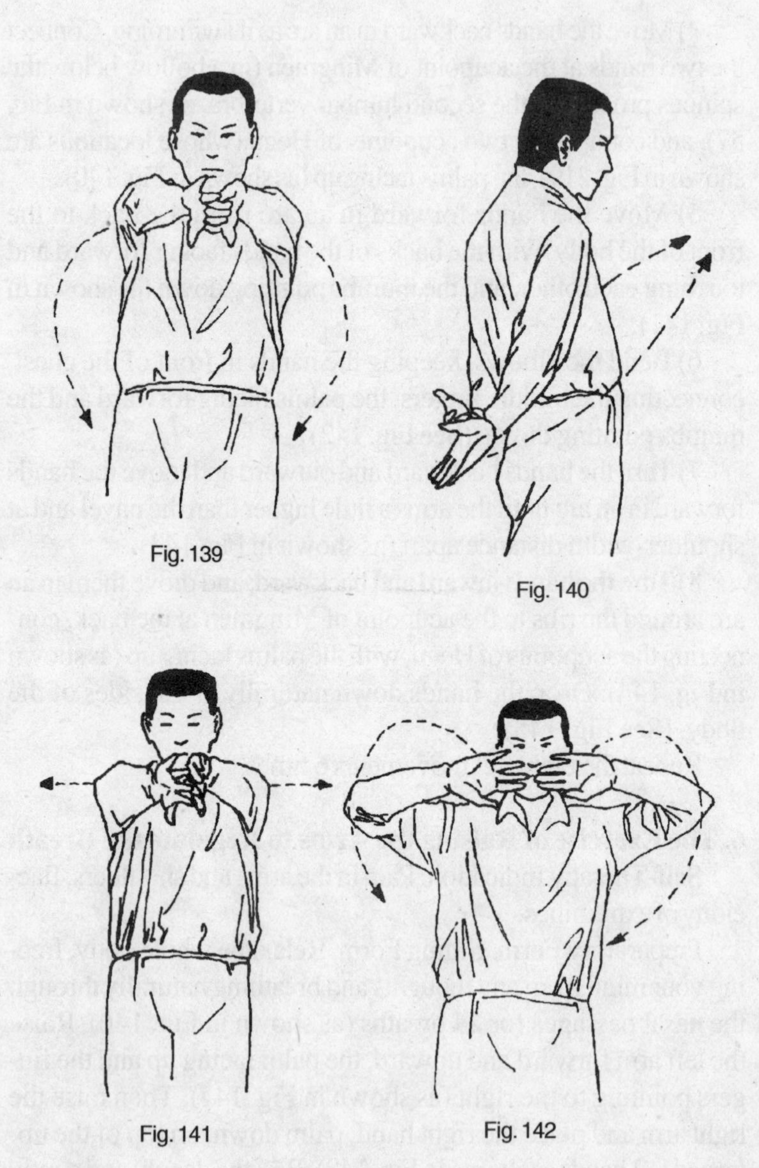

Fig. 139

Fig. 140

Fig. 141

Fig. 142

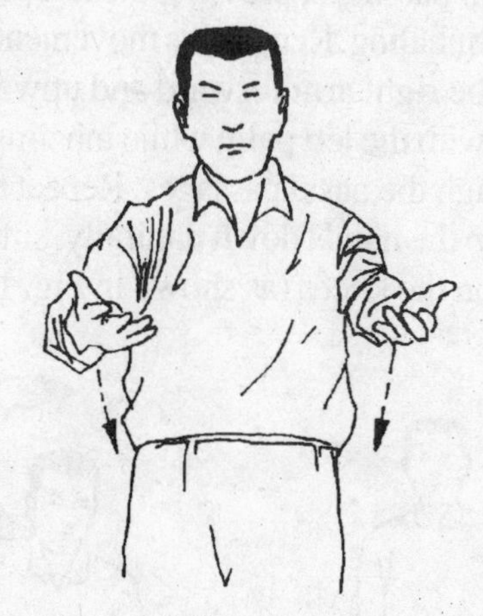

Fig. 143

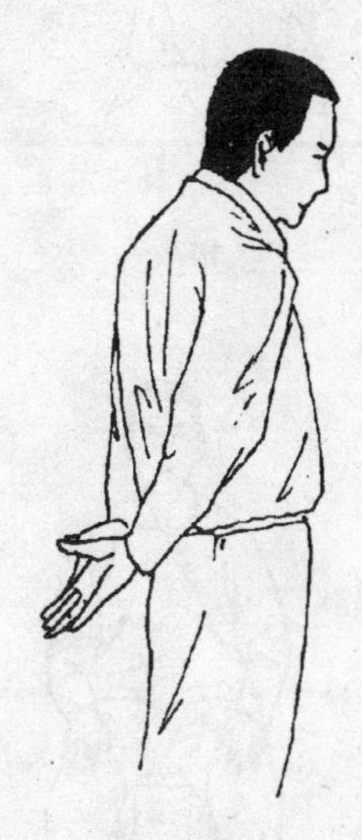

Fig. 144

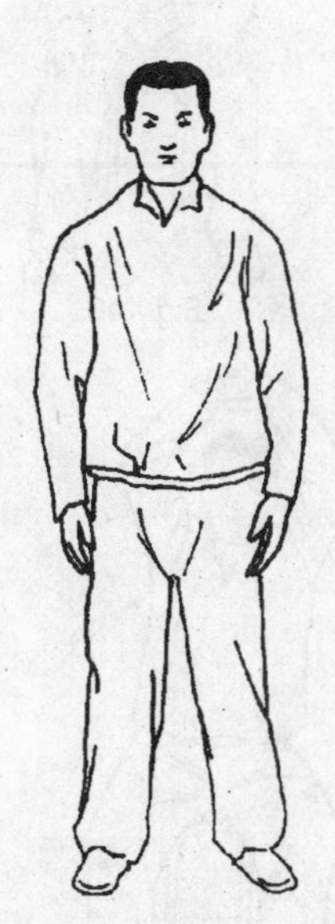

Fig. 145

through the nasal passages, pressing the left palm hard with the right palm while inhaling. Repeat this movement 12 times.

Then raise the right arm forward and upward, and press the right palm hard with the left palm while inhaling. Breathe deeply and gently through the nasal passages. Repeat the movement 12 times. Then drop the hands down naturally, sitting for 5 minutes with the hands on the knees (as shown in Fig. 149).

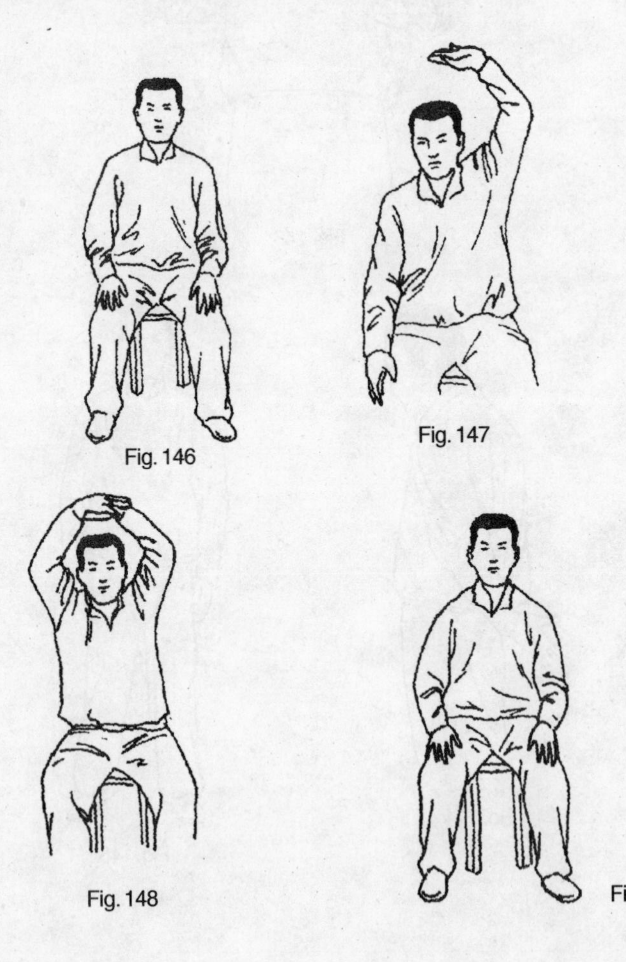

Fig. 146

Fig. 147

Fig. 148

Fig. 149

7. The Exercise of Irradiating the Acupoints of Jienue with the Qi

Self-Therapy Indication: Malaria and pain moving about the chest and hypochondria.

Preparatory Form: Standing Form (2). Relax the whole body. Bend the knees slightly, the hands closing in front of the chest. Keep the eyes nearly closed, looking at the tips of the middle fingers for 5 minutes (as shown in Fig. 150). Direct the two palms to the two acupoints of Jienue (4 cun right below the right and the left breasts in the chest, as shown in Fig. 152), the distance between the hands and the chest being 10 cm. Irradiate the acupoints for 20 minutes (as shown in Fig. 151).

8. The Exercise of Bending the Trunk Forward and Backward

Self-Therapy Indication: This exercise can regulate the five internal organs, and cure lumbago and backache.

Kneel down on a hard bed (as shown in Fig. 153). Stretch the arms forward and support the trunk with the arms (as shown in Fig. 154). Bend the left elbow and support the left side of the body with the left elbow. Turn the left ribs, the left side of the waist and the left hip leftward and downward, lying on the left side of the body (as shown in Fig. 155). Imagine that the Qi is dispersing around the lower back. Then bend the right elbow, supporting the right side of the body with the right elbow. Turn the right ribs, the right side of the waist and the right hip rightward and downward, lying on the right side of the body. Imagine that the Qi is dispersing around the lower back. Repeat the left-turning and the right-turning 6 times.

Then kneel still on the hard bed. Raise the hands over the head and bend the hands and the trunk backward, feeling that a current of cold air is being discharged from the spine. Bend the trunk backward in this way 12 times. (See Fig. 156)

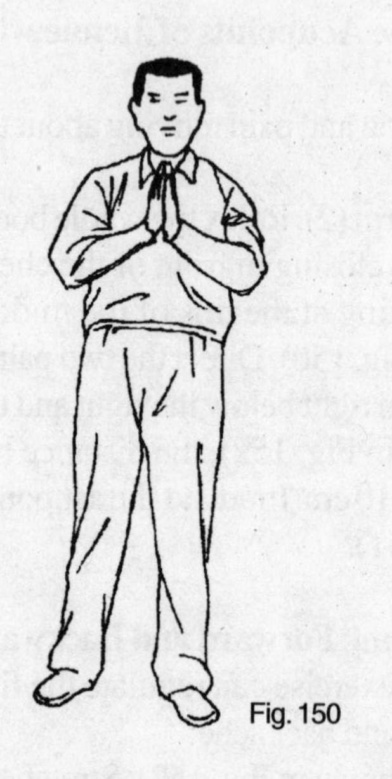
Fig. 150

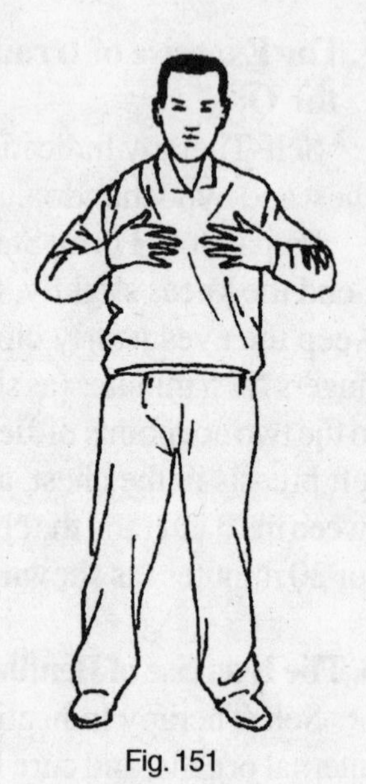
Fig. 151

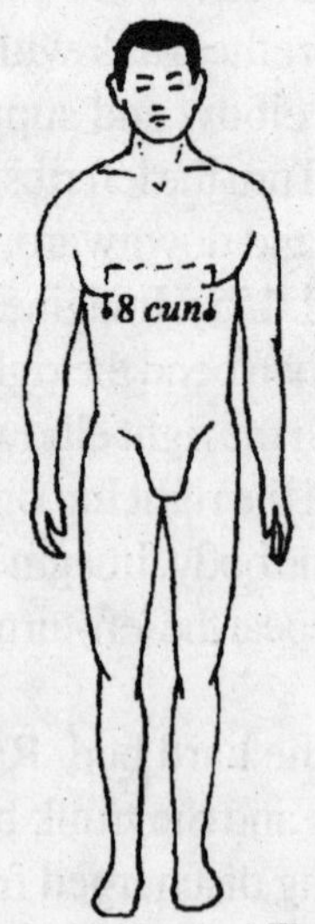

Fig. 152

9. The Exercise of Turning the Waist to Move the Qi

Self-Therapy Indication: Pain in the waist, kidneys and hypochondria.

Preparatory Form: Standing Form (2). Relax the whole body, with the eyes looking forward and the hands hanging down naturally. Stand still for 5 to 10 minutes, freeing the mind from any thoughts (as shown in Fig. 157). Move the hands from the sides to the front of the chest, the forearms kept horizontal, and the hands closed and pushing on each other (as shown in Fig. 158). Turn the trunk to the left as far as possible, with the eyes following the hands while raising the closed hands over the head (as shown in Fig.159 and Fig. 160). Inhale slowly through the nasal passages while turning and begin to exhale while stretching the arms. Move the hands to the front of the chest, turning the trunk to the former standing form (as shown in Fig. 161). Visualise the acupoints of Baihui, Yintang, Renzhong, Danzhong, Middle Dantian, Huiyin, Fengshi, Yanglingquan, Xuanzhong, Yongquan, Sanyinjiao, Yinlingquan, Xuehai, Huiyin, Mingmen, and along the middle line at the back up to the acupoint of Baihui at the top of the head. (See Fig. 162)

Turn the trunk to the right as far as possible, with the eyes following the hands while raising the closed hands over the head (as shown in Fig. 163 and Fig. 164). Inhale slowly through the nasal passages while turning and begin to exhale while stretching the arms. Move the hands to the front of the chest, turning the trunk back to the former standing form (as shown in Fig. 165). Then visualise the acupoints mentioned above (as shown in Fig. 162). Repeat the left and right turning 6 times.

Closing Form: Separate the little fingers, the third, the middle, the forefingers and the thumbs, respectively. Keep the hands down naturally by the sides of the thigh. (See Fig. 166)

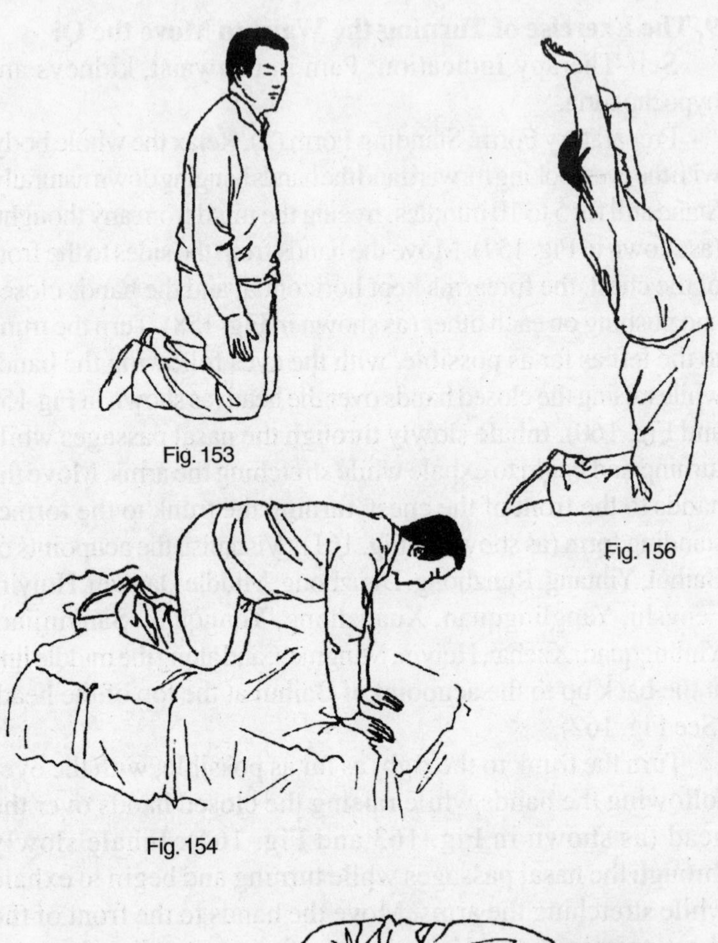

Fig. 153

Fig. 156

Fig. 154

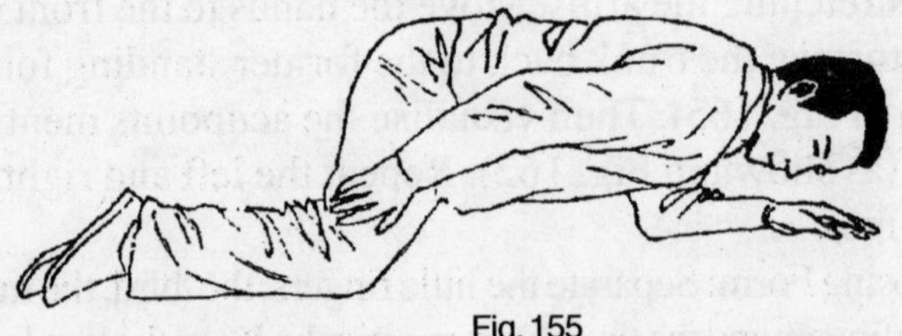

Fig. 155

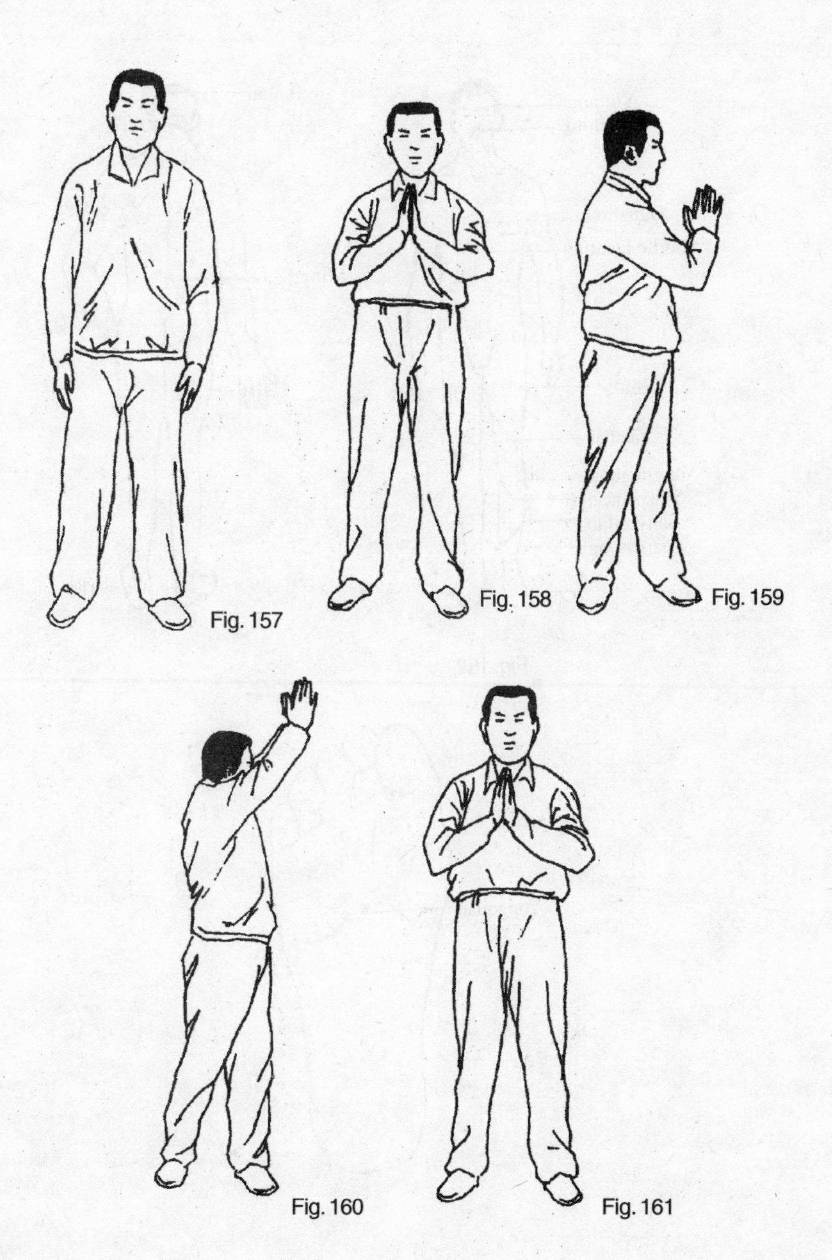

Fig. 157 Fig. 158 Fig. 159

Fig. 160 Fig. 161

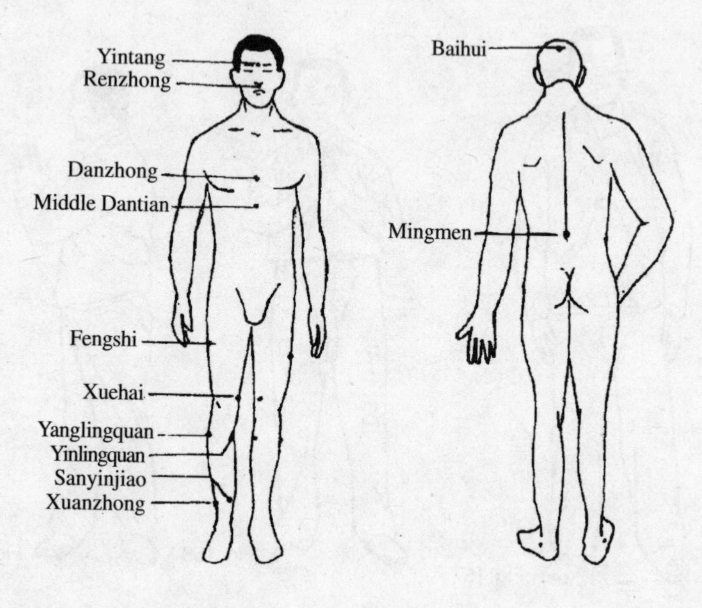
Yintang
Renzhong
Danzhong
Middle Dantian
Fengshi
Xuehai
Yanglingquan
Yinlingquan
Sanyinjiao
Xuanzhong
Baihui
Mingmen

Fig. 162

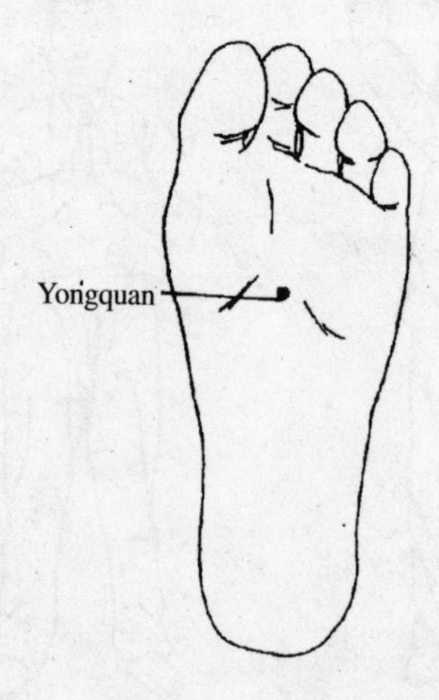
Yongquan

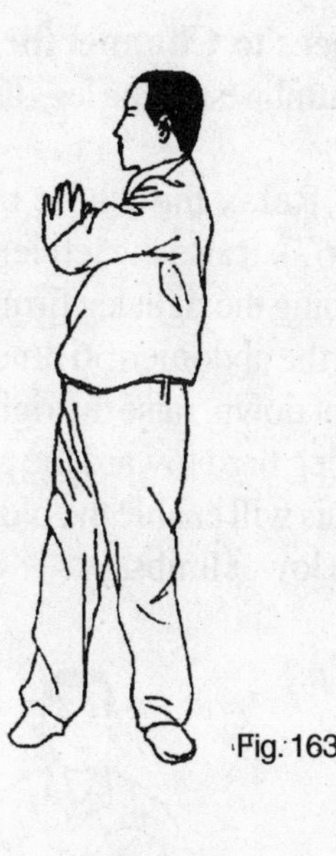

Fig. 163

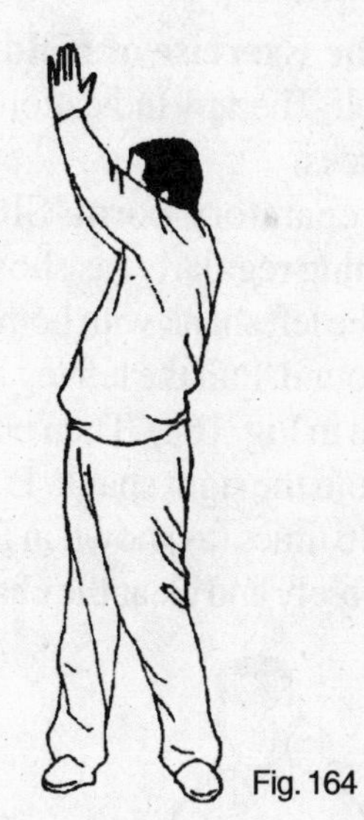

Fig. 164

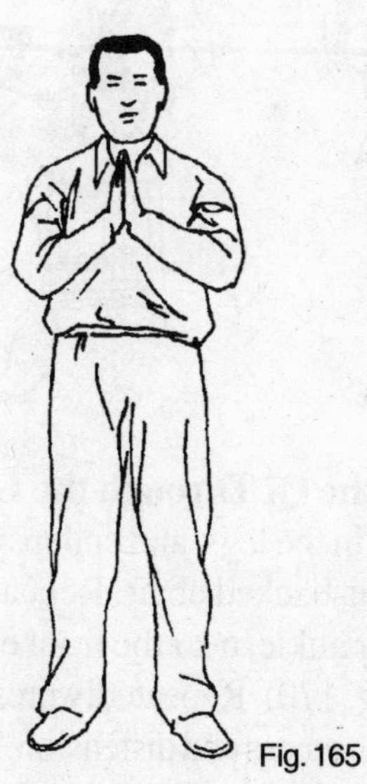

Fig. 165

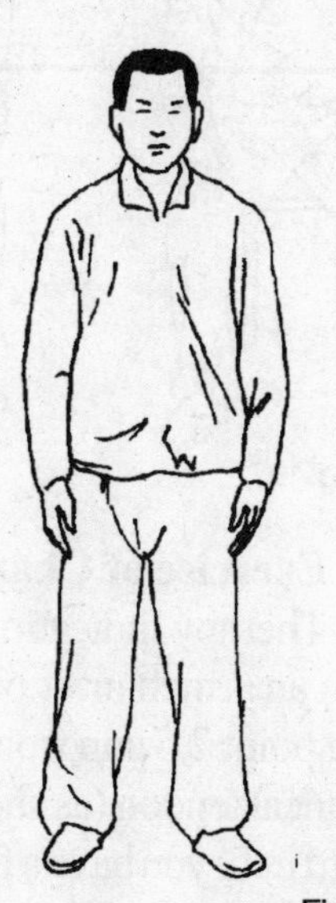

Fig. 166

10. The Exercise of Holding the Knees to Channel the Qi

Self-Therapy Indication: Pain and numbness in the legs below the knees.

Preparatory Form: Sitting Form. Relax the whole body, breathing regularly (as shown in Fig. 167). Raise the left leg and hold the left shank with both hands, keeping the right leg firmly on the ground. Pull the left leg hard toward the abdomen 36 times (as shown in Fig. 168). Then put the left foot down, raise the right leg and hold the right shank. Pull the right leg hard toward the abdomen 36 times (as shown in Fig. 169). This will enable the blood to flow freely and clear the channels in the lower limbs.

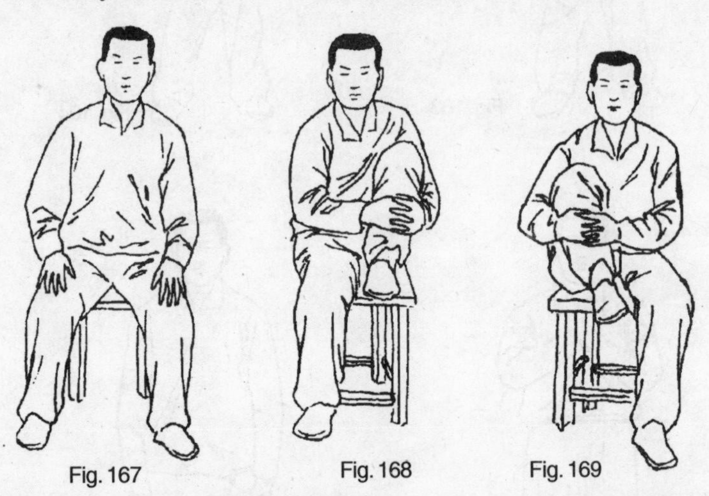

Fig. 167 Fig. 168 Fig. 169

11. The Exercise of Channelling the Qi Through the Legs

Self-Therapy Indication: Edema in the legs, and epilepsy.

Sit in an armchair or on a straight-backed chair. Repeatedly press the point 2.5 cun from the inner ankle, near the front end of the calcaneal tendon (as shown in Fig. 170). Repeatedly press the point hard until you have a feeling of soreness and distension. Then rub the point up and down with your hands 108 times. Do the

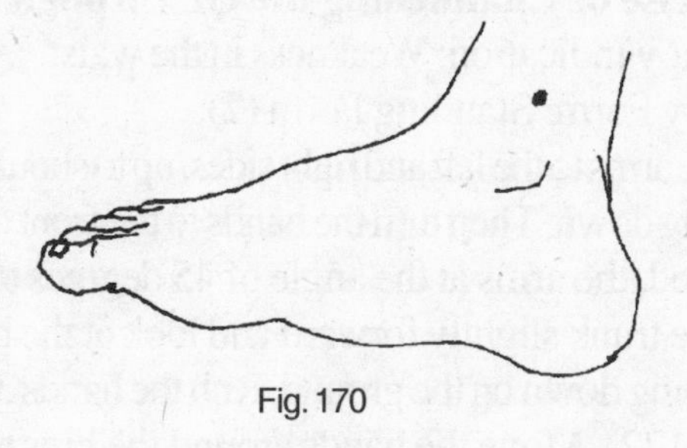
Fig. 170

exercise every morning and evening.

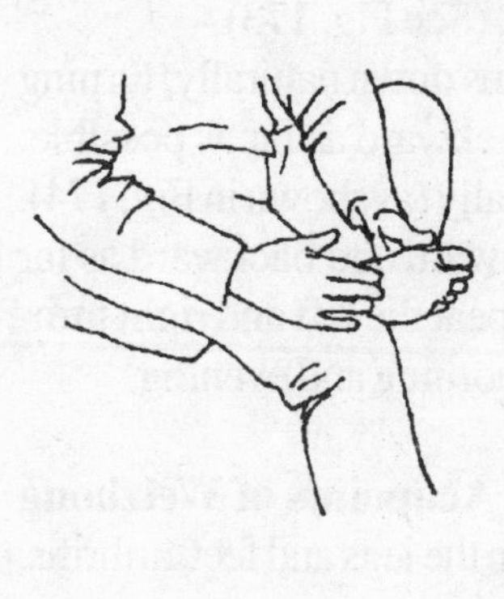

12. The Exercise of Massaging the Feet

Self-Therapy Indication: Weakness in the lower limbs.

Sit on a bed or in an armchair. Bend the left foot and hold the left toes with the left hand, rubbing the sole of the foot with the right hand using a little force 108 times. Then rub the sole of the right foot in the same way as described above (as shown in Fig. 171).

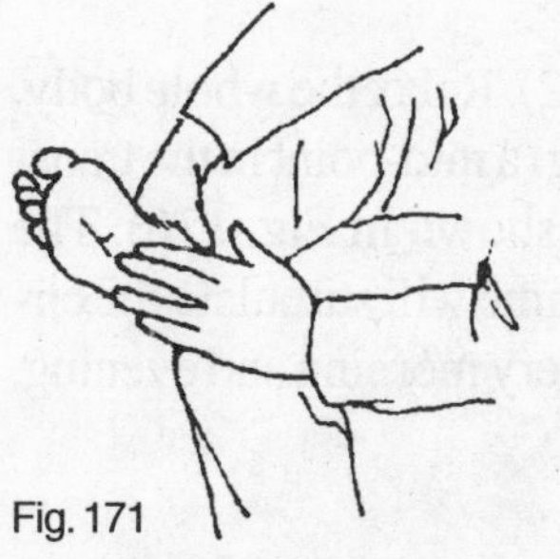
Fig. 171

Then rub big toes against the second toes. Keep them rubbing each other 36 times at the beginng and 108 times when you get used to the rubbing. Do the two sets of the movements mentioned above every morning and evening.

The movement of the feet is the key to the whole body because all the channels of the body meet in the feet.

13. The Exercise of Channelling the Qi Through the Waist

Self-Therapy Indication: Weakness in the waist.

Preparatory Form: Standing Form (2).

1) Raise the arms to the left and right sides, up to shoulder-height, the palms facing down. Then turn the hands to the front of the body, the hands closed, the arms at the angle of 45 degrees to the upper trunk. Bend the trunk slightly forward and look at the hands, with your toes pressing down on the ground. Rub the hands 36 times (as shown in Fig. 172). Move the hands around the hips to the back, with the palms touching the acupoints of Shenshu (1.5 cun lateral below the spinous process of the second lumbar vertebra). Rub the acupoints up and down 36 to 64 times. (See Fig. 173)

2) Standing Form (2). Hang the arms down naturally, turning the head and the trunk leftward and backward as far as possible, with the arms following the trunk naturally (as shown in Fig. 174). Then turn the head and the trunk rightward and backward as far as possible (as shown in Fig. 175). Repeat the left and right turning 108 times. Do the exercise every morning and evening.

14. The Exercise of Visualising the Acupoints of Weizhong

Self-Therapy Indication: Cramps in the legs and feet, arthritis, and leg paralysis.

Preparatory Form: Standing Form (2). Relax the whole body.

Visualise the acupoints of Weizhong (a mid-point in the transverse line at the back of the knees, as shown in Fig. 176). The performance of this exercise for a long time will stimulate the circulation of the blood. Do the exercise every morning and evening, and each time for at least 20 minutes.

15. The Exercise of Relaxing the Kness and Ankles

Self-Therapy Indication: Arthritis, articular rheumatism, pain in the ankle joints and numbness in the legs.

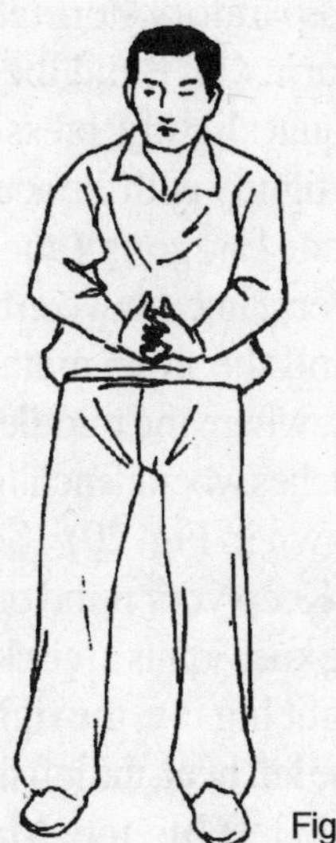
Fig. 172

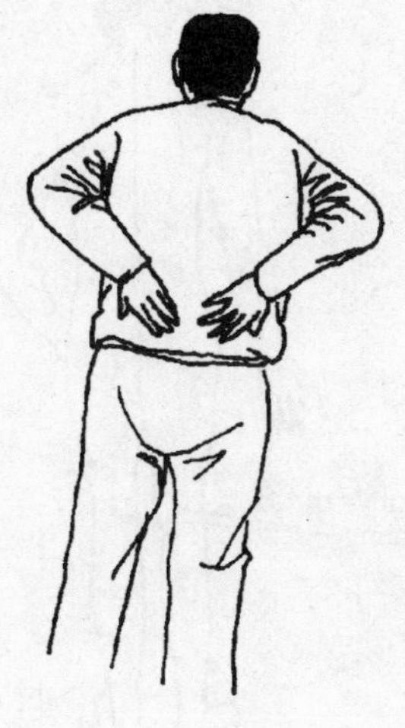
Fig. 173

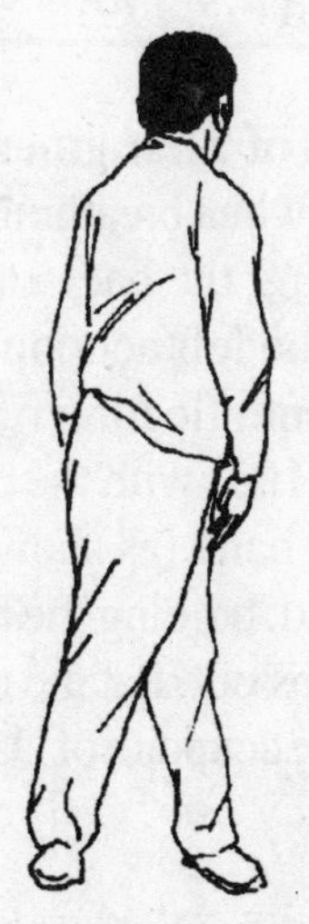
Fig. 174

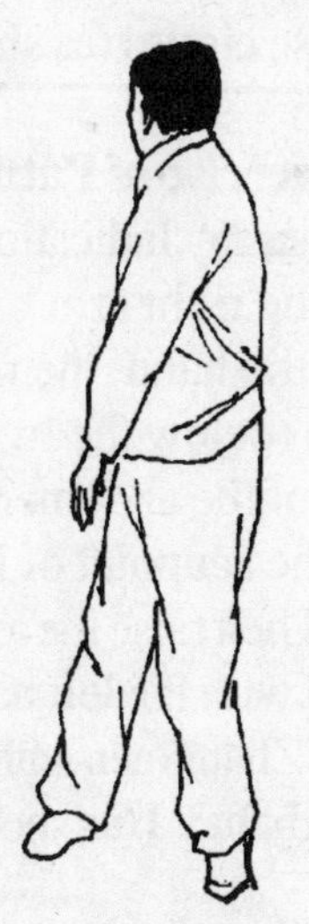
Fig. 175

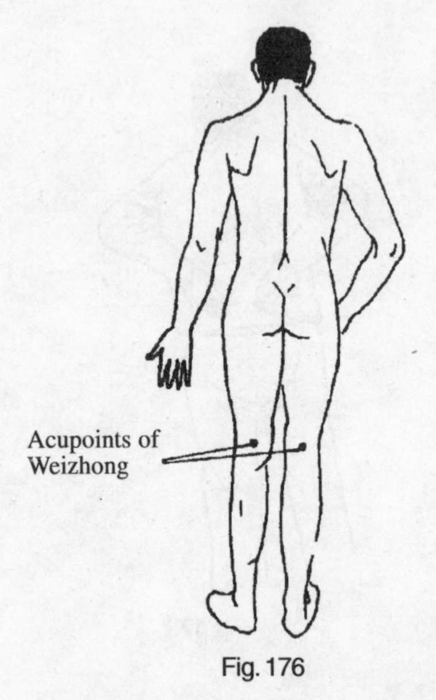

Fig. 176

Preparatory Form: Standing Form (1). Bend the knees and squat slightly, pressing the knees tightly with the acupoints of Inner Laogong (above the transverse line, between the second and the third metacarpal bones, where the middle finger tip touches when clenching a fist, as shown in Fig. 20). (See Fig. 177). Keep your mind on moving the knee joints in circle along the right big toe, the right little toe, the left heel, the left little toe and the left big toe. Make 36 clockwise circles and 36 counterclockwise circles (as shown in Fig. 178 and Fig. 179).

16. The Exercise of Patting the Acupoints of Zhangmen

Self-Therapy Indication: Pain in the chest when breathing.

Raise the right arm over the head, holding the back of the head with the hand, the right ribs out. Pat the left acupoint of Zhangmen (below the free ends of the eleventh floating ribs at both sides of the abdomen, as shown in Fig. 103) with the right hand and the acupoint of Dabao with the left hand (as shown in Fig. 180). Then raise the left arm over the head, holding the back of the head with the left hand, with the left ribs out. Pat the right acupoint of Zhangmen with the left hand and the acupoint of Dabao with the right hand (as shown in Fig. 181).

17. The Exercise of Breathing to Allay a Fever

Self-Therapy Indication: A fever caused by internal injury.

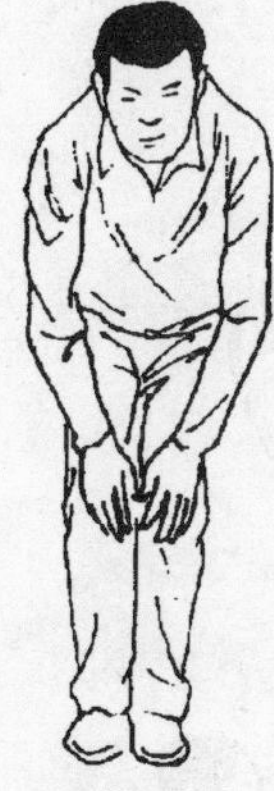

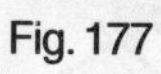
Fig. 177

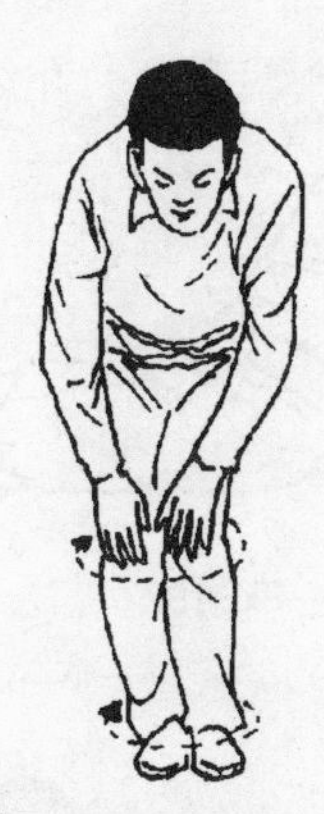

Fig. 178

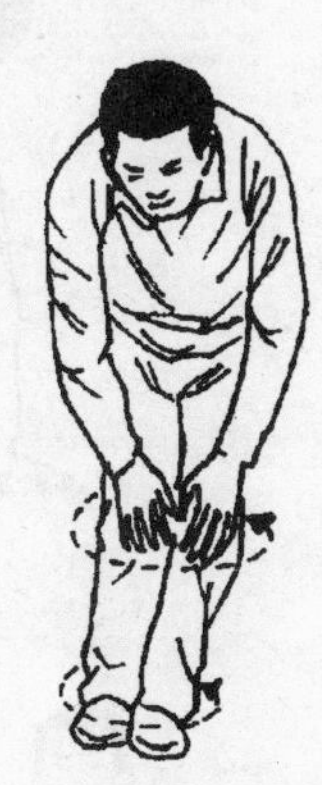

Fig. 179

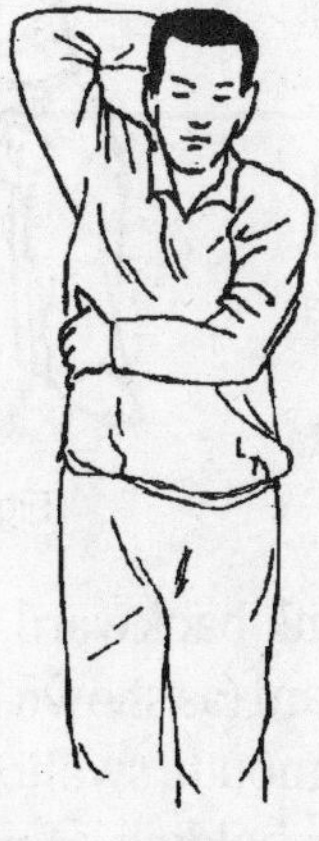

Fig. 180

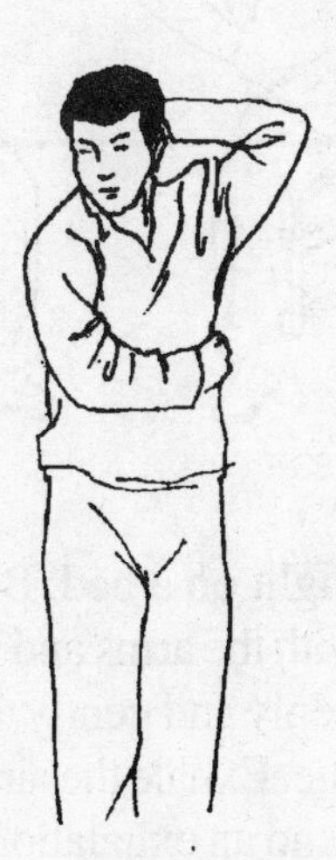

Fig. 181

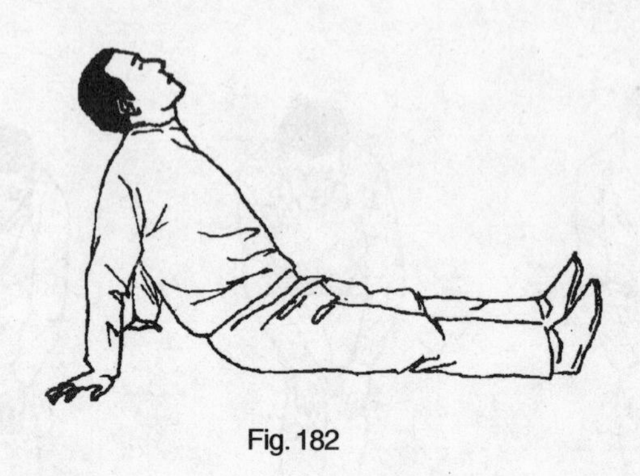

Fig. 182

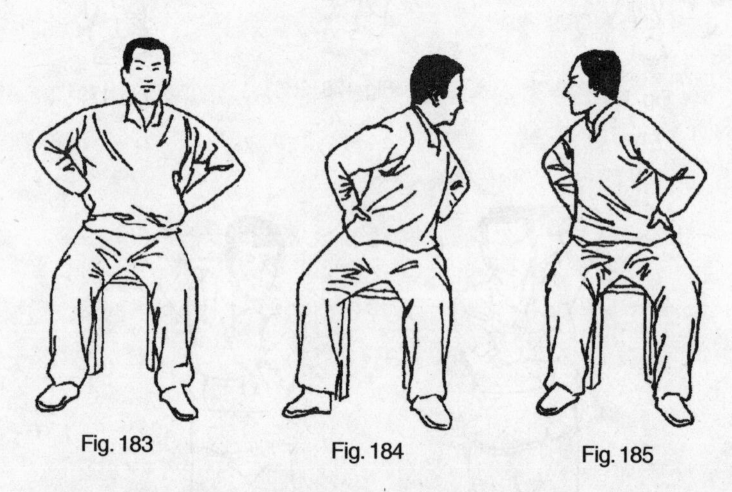

Fig. 183 Fig. 184 Fig. 185

Sit upright on a bed. Bend the trunk backward, supporting the trunk with the arms and facing upward (as shown in Fig. 182). Breathe deeply and gently through the mouth, swallowing the air as you inhale. Exhale the air slowly after holding it for a while. An inhalation and an exhalation make up one cycle, which should be repeated 64 times.

18. The Exercise of Turning the Trunk to Channel the Qi

Self-therapy Indication: Abdomen affected by cold, and stuffy chest.

Preparapory Form: Sitting Form. Sit upright, relaxing the whole body, the hands on the hips, the thumbs pointing forward, and the other fingers pointing backwards (as shown in Fig. 183). Draw in the chest and the shoulders, turning the trunk to the left as far as possible (as shown in Fig. 184). Then turn the trunk to the right as far as possible (as shown in Fig. 185). The left-turning and right-turning make up one cycle, which should be repeated 64 times.

CHAPTER IX THE FIVE SENSE ORGANS (EYES, TEETH, EARS, NOSE AND THROAT)

1. The Exercise of Lying on the Stomach to Channel the Qi

Self-Therapy Indication: Diseases in the nine orifices (the five sense organs and the urethra and the anus), and weakness and cold in the lower limbs.

Lie on your stomach on a hard bed, with your feet straight and close together (as shown in Fig. 186). Bend the knees, until the heels touch the hips. Stretch your arms backward, holding the feet with your hands and pulling them upward, with the chest out and the neck bending backward. Pull the feet 36 times (as shown in Fig. 187).

2. The Exercise of Irradiating and Pressing the Eyes

Self-Therapy Indication: Ophthalmocopia.

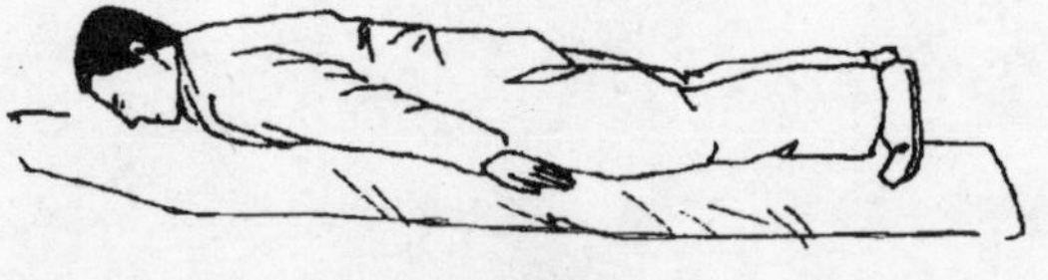

Fig. 186

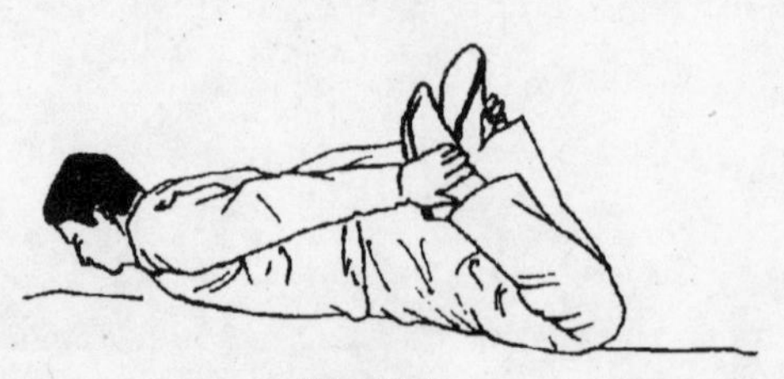

Fig. 187

Preparatory Form: Standing Form (2). At daybreak, rub the hands 36 times until they are warm. (If it is cold outside, do the exercise indoors or soak the hands in hot water before rubbing them together). Then close the eyes slightly. Cover the eyes tightly with the palms after rubbing the acupoints of Laogong (above the transverse line, between the second and the third metacarpal bones, where the middle finger tip touches when clenching a fist, as shown in Fig. 20). Breathe naturally 36 times (as shown in Fig. 188). Then press the eyeballs gently with the forefingers and middle fingers 36 times. (See Fig. 189).

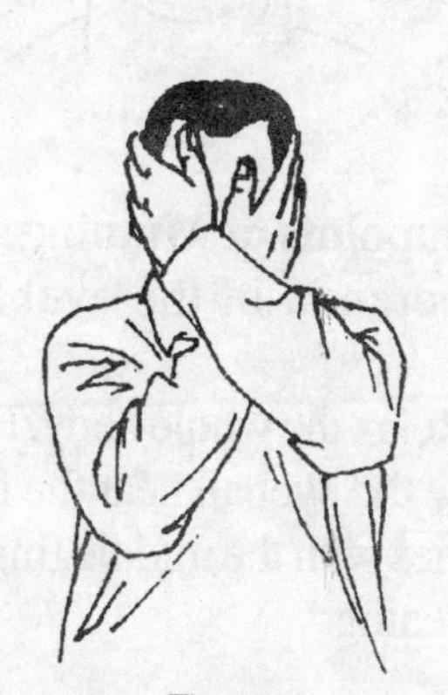

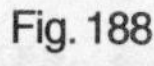

Fig. 188

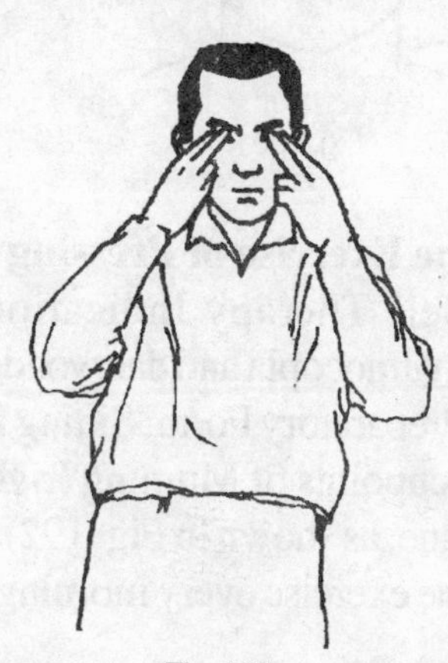

Fig. 189

3. The Exercise of Rubbing the Acupoints of Upper Yingxiang

Self-Therapy Indication: Epiphora induced by wind.

Preparatory Form: Sitting Form. Relax the whole body. Press the acupounts of Upper Yingxiang (0.5 cun below the inner canthi, besides the root of the nose, as shown in Fig. 190) with the two middle fingers 108 times. Do the exercise every morning and evening.

4. The Exercise of Pressing the Lower End of the Nasal Septum

Self-Therapy Indication: Xerophthalmia and ophthalmia.

Lie on your back. Press the lower end of the nasal septum (as shown in Fig. 191) 108 times with the thumb. Do the exercise every morning and evening.

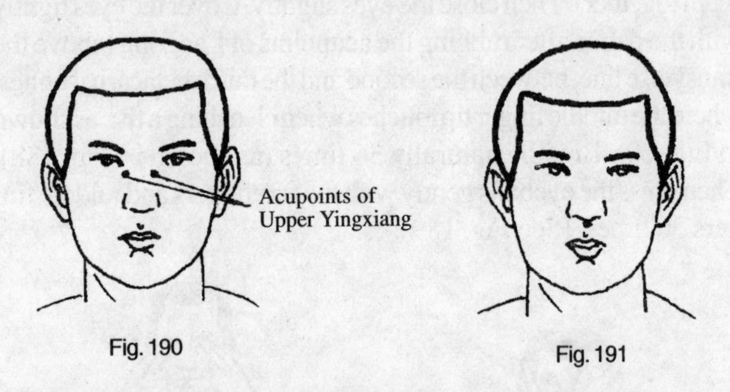

Fig. 190

Fig. 191

5. The Exercise of Pressing the Acupoints of Muming

Self-Therapy Indication: Hyperemia in the eyeballs, ophthalmocopia and dacryoadenitis.

Preparatory Form: Sitting Form. Relax the whole body. Press the acupoints of Muming (right above the eyeball near the front hairline, as shown in Fig. 192) 108 times with the middle fingers. Do the exercise every morning and evening.

6. The Exercise of Visualising the Acupoint of Yintang

Self-Therapy Indication: Glaucoma, temporary nearsightedness and cataract.

Preparatory Form: Standing Form (2). Relax the whole body. Visualise the acupoint of Yintang between the eyebrows (as shown in Fig. 193) and relax the acupoint while visualising it in case you feel dizzy.

7. The Exercise of Irradiating and Turning the Eyeballs

Self-Therapy Indication: Nearsightedness.

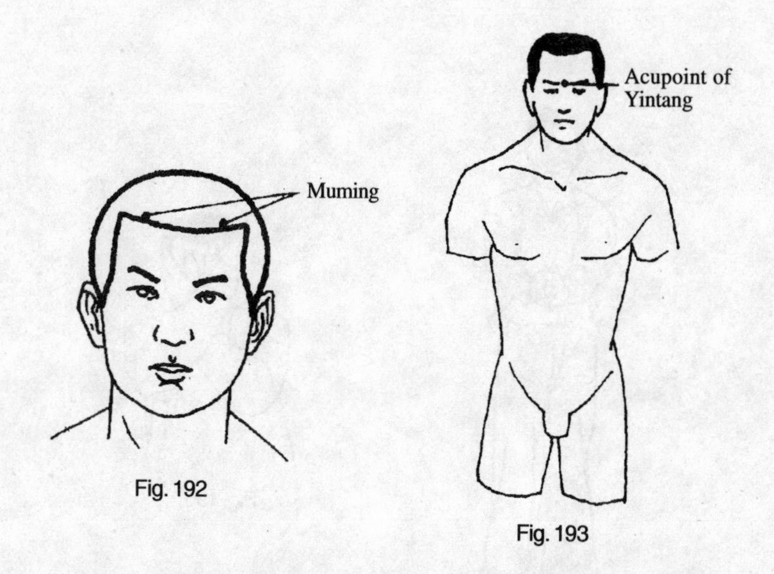

Fig. 192

Fig. 193

Preparatory Form: Standing Form (2). Relax the whole body. Stretch the arms to the left and right, moving the hands upward and forward in an arc, with the hands closed in front of the chest (as shown in Fig. 194). Fix your mind on the centre of each palm for 2 minutes before rubbing the hands 108 times. Cover the right eye with the left hand, and the left eye with the right hand (as shown in Fig. 195) with the eyeballs making 18 clockwise rotations and 18 counterclockwise rotations. Put the hands down and look at an object in the distance for about 20 seconds before closing the eyes. Repeat the exercise 3 times.

8. The Exercise of Washing and Turning the Eyeballs

Self-Therapy Indication: Farsightedness and presbyopia.

Preparatory Form: Standing Form (2). Rub the hands 108 times. Cover the right eye with the left hand and the left eye with the right hand, the eyeballs making 18 clockwise and 18 counterclockwise rotations before closing them for 5 minutes. (See Fig. 196).

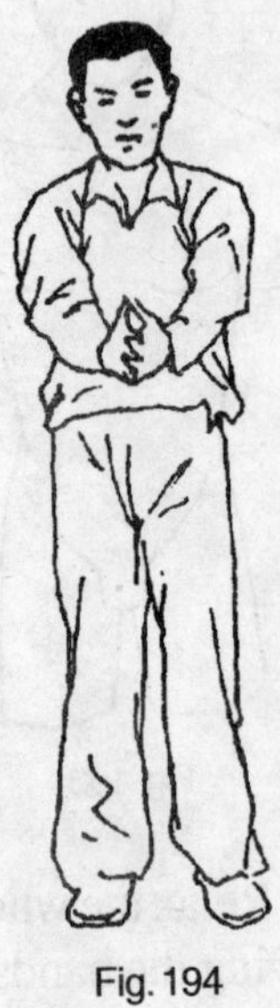

Fig. 194

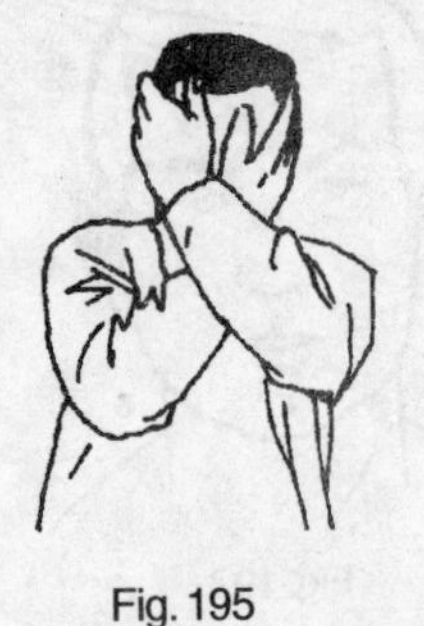

Fig. 195

Take a half basin of clean water and put your face into the water (as shown in Fig. 197). Open the eyes slowly, the eyeballs making 36 clockwise rotations and 36 counterclockwise rotations.

9. The Exercise of Irradiating and Washing the Eyes

Self-Therapy Indication: Cataract and early glaucoma.

Preparatory Form: Standing Form (2). Relax the whole body. Rub the hands 64 times. Move the hands backward, pressing the acupoints of Shenshu (1.5 cun and lateral below the spinous process of the second lumbar vertebra) with the acupoints of Laogong (above the transverse line, between the second and the third metacarpal bones, where the middle finger tip touches when clenching a fist, as shown in Fig. 20) and rubbing the acupoints up and down.

An up and down rubbing makes one cycle. Repeat the cycle 64 times (as shown in Fig. 198). Then cover the eyes with the acupoints of Laogong (as shown in Fig. 199), the eyeballs making 6 clockwise rotations and 6 counterclockwise rotations. Repeat the eyeball's turning 6 times. After that, make each palm a hollow and massage the rim of each eye up and down with the hollow palms 36 times and another 36 times in the opposite direction.

Take a basin of clean water every morning, put your face into it, and open your eyes slowly, the eyes making 36 clockwise rotations and 36 counterclockwise rotations. (See Fig. 197)

10. The Exercise of Holding the Knees to Channel the Qi

Self-Therapy Indication: Epiphora induced by wind, and numbness in the lower limbs.

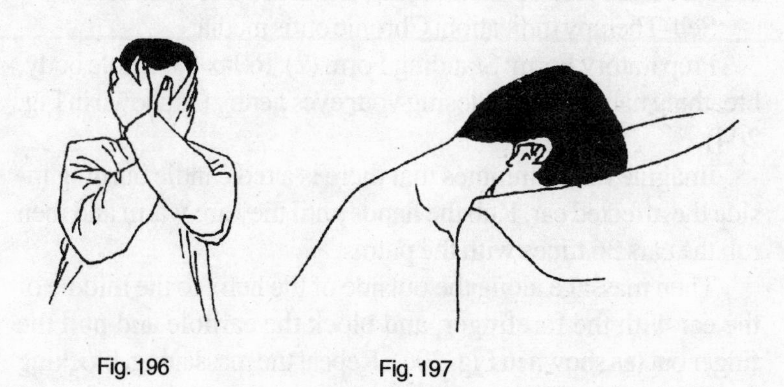

Fig. 196 Fig. 197

Sit on a hard bed, separating your legs, with the knees bent slightly outward, and resting your hands on the knees (as shown in Fig. 200). Close the eyes gently and breathe naturally 36 times. Draw the left knee backward, holding it with your hands. Stretch the right leg, turning the instep outward until it touches the surface of the bed (as shown in Fig. 201). Inhale deeply and gently, drawing in as much air as you can through the nasal passages before exhaling. Breathe in this way 7 times. Then hold the right knee with your hands, stretching the left leg and turning the left instep outward until it touches the surface of the bed (as shown in Fig. 202). Inhale deeply and gently through the nasal passages before exhaling. Breathe in this way 7 times. Finally return to the former sitting form, breathing for 3 to 5 minutes and conclude the exercise (as shown in Fig. 203).

11. The Exercise of Visualising the Inside of the Ears

Self-Therapy Indication: Chronic otitis media.

Preparatory Form: Standing Form (2). Relax the whole body, breathing naturally and closing your eyes gently (as shown in Fig. 204).

Imagine for 20 minutes that there is a red candle burning inside the affected ear. Rub the hands until they are warm and then rub the ears 36 times with the palms.

Then massage along the outside of the helix to the middle of the ear with the forefinger, and block the earhole and pull the finger out (as shown in Fig. 206). Repeat the massaging, blocking and pulling 6 times.

12. The Exercise of Rubbing the Ears to Preserve the Fervor of Youth

Self-Therapy Indication: Deficiency of kidney Qi, tinnitus, and pain in the ears.

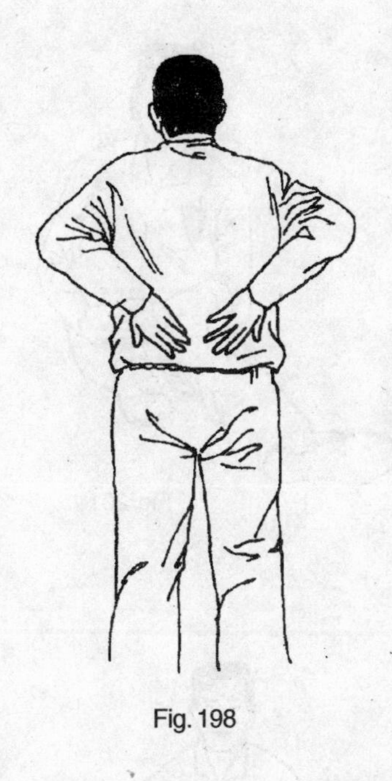

Fig. 198

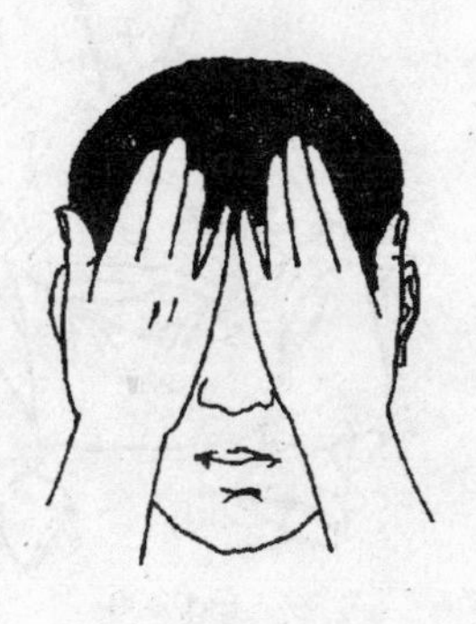

Fig. 199

Preparatory Form: Standing Form (2). Relax the whole body, rubbing your hands until they are warm. Rub the ears and the skin around the ears so as to keep the Qi and the blood circulating fully there. Rub the ears until they are warm (as shown in Fig. 207). Then stretch the two forefingers, inserting them into the earholes and blocking the external auditory meatuses. Then withdraw the forefingers quickly. Repeat the inserting and withdrawing of the forefingers 6 times. (See Fig. 208)

13. The Exercise of Pressing the Acupoints of Biliu

Self-Therapy Indication: Stuffy nose, and persistent nasal

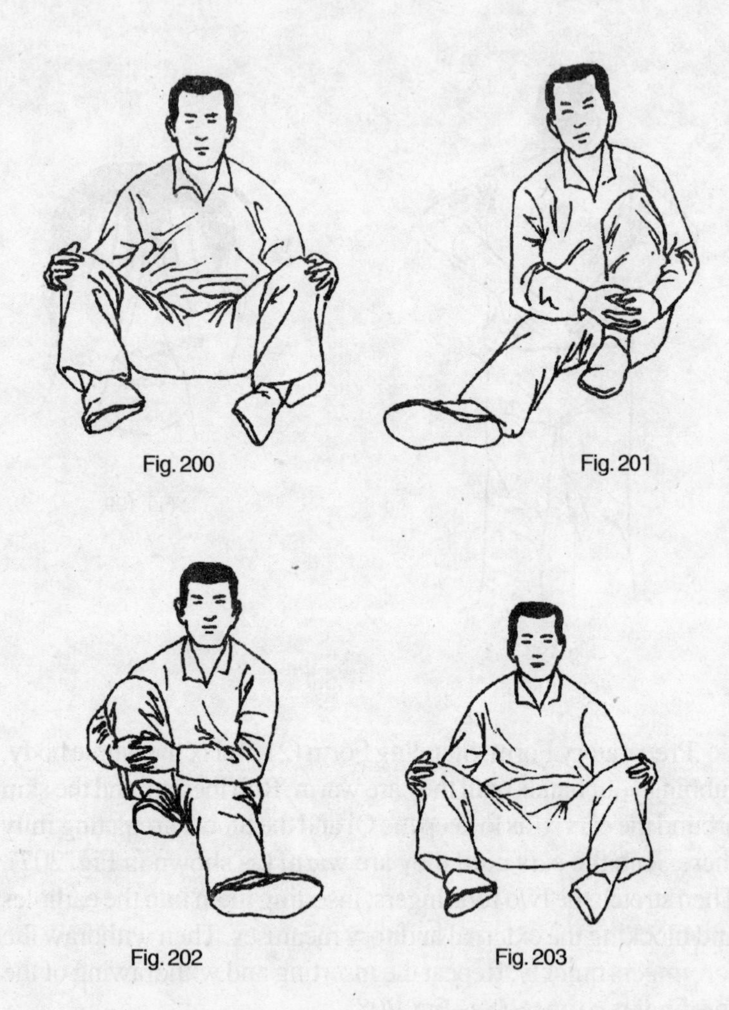

Fig. 200 Fig. 201 Fig. 202 Fig. 203

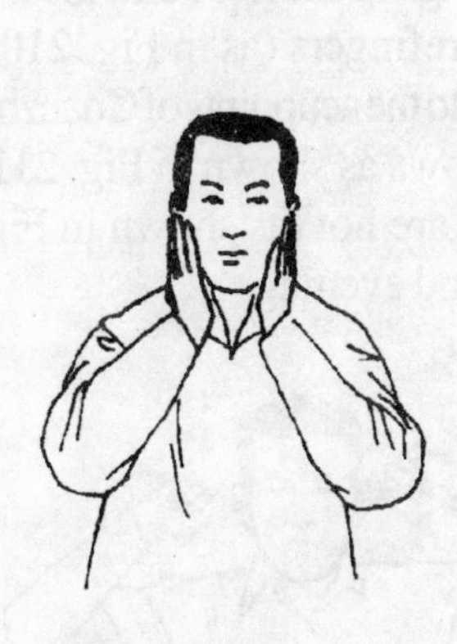

Fig. 205

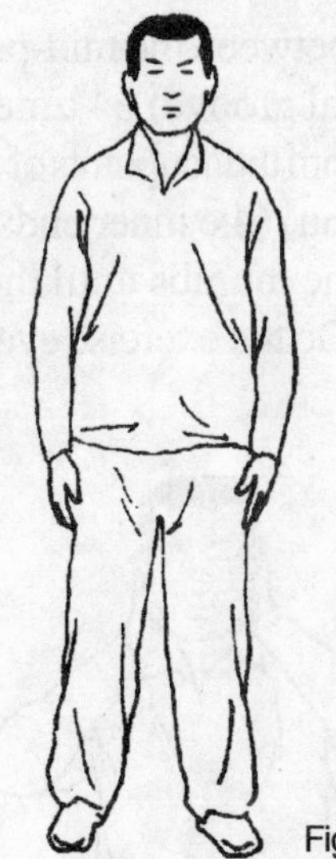

Fig. 204

discharge.

Preparatory Form: Sitting Form. Sit upright and be relaxed. Put the right thumb and the right forefinger below the nostrils, repeatedly pressing the two acupoints of Biliu between the nasal septum and the wings of the nose (as shown in Fig. 209). Press the acupoints with moderate force 64 times, and press them every other hour until you feel better.

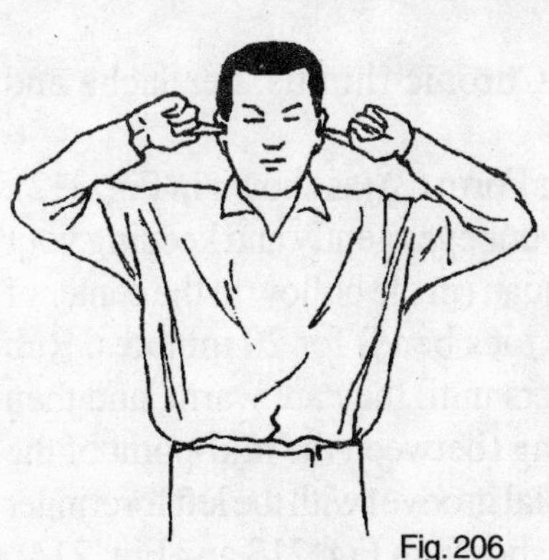

Fig. 206

14. The Exercise of Massaging the Acupoints of Yingxiang

Self-Therapy Indication: Rhinitis.

Preparatory Form: Standing Form (2). Massage the acupoints of Yingxiang (a point between the mid-point of the wings of the nose and the nasolabial groove) 64 times with the forefingers (as in Fig. 210). Rub from the acupoints of Yingxiang up to the acupoints of Cuanzhu (Zanzhu) (the inner ends of the eyebrows as shown in Fig. 211) with the thumbs until the nose wings are hot (as shown in Fig. 276). Do the exercise every morning and evening

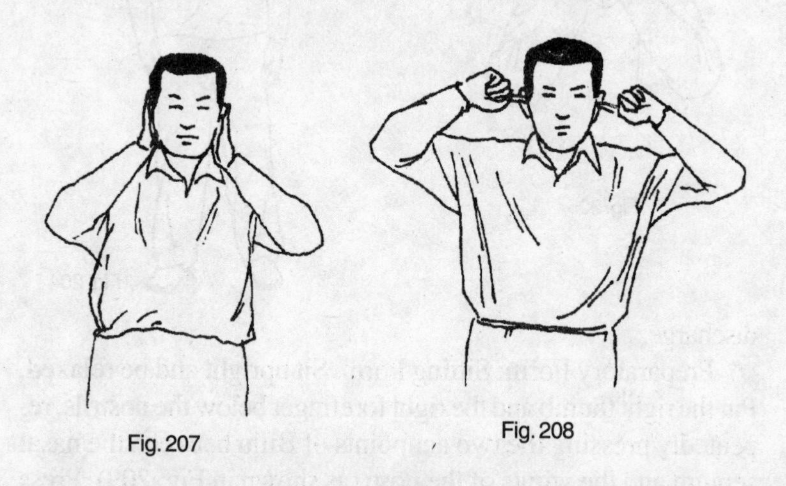

Fig. 207 Fig. 208

15. The Exercise of Channelling the Qi Through the Acupoints of Yongquan

Self-Therapy Indication: Chronic rhinitis, headache and dizziness.

Preparatory Form: Standing Form (2) (as shown in Fig. 212). Relax the whole body, closing your eyes gently and keeping your mind on the acupoints of Yongquan (in the hollow in the center of the sole of each foot when the toes bend) for 20 minutes. Rub your palms with your forefingers until they are warm, and then press the acupoints of Yingxiang (between the mid-point of the wing of the nose and the nasolabial groove) with the left forefinger first and then with the right (as shown in Fig. 213 and Fig. 214).

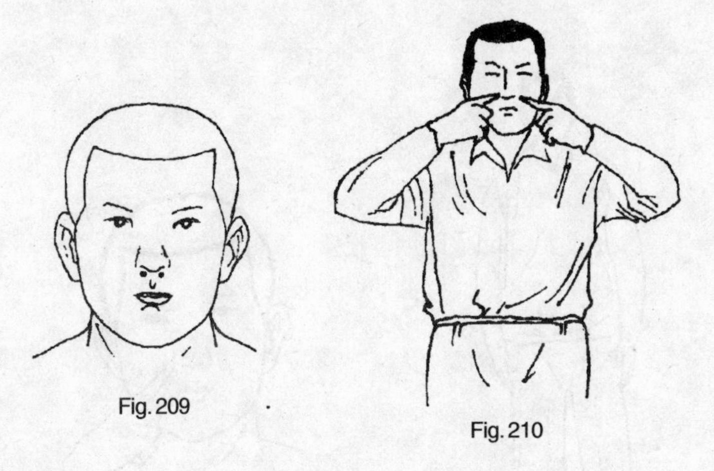

Fig. 209

Fig. 210

Rub each side 108 times. Do the exercise every morning and evening.

16. The Exercise of Pressing the Nose to Clear the Nasal Passages

Self-Therapy Indication: Stuffy nose, and deficiency of olfaction.

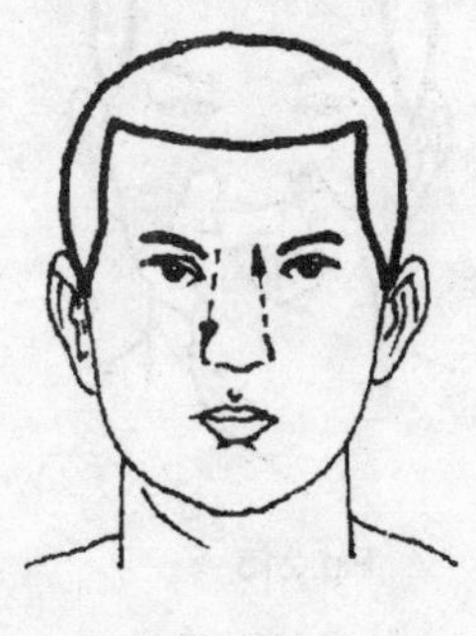

Fig. 211

Preparatory Form: Siting Form. Sit facing the sun and be relaxed. Hold the breath 3 times before massaging the wings of the nose until the area is hot. Do the exercise 2 to 3 times daily (as shown in Fig. 215).

17. The Exercise of Visualising the Acupoint of Fengfu

Self-Therapy Indication: Headache, epitaxis, pharyngitis.

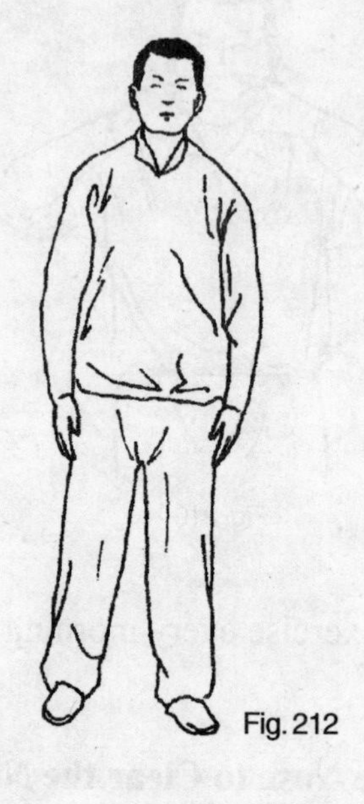

Fig. 212

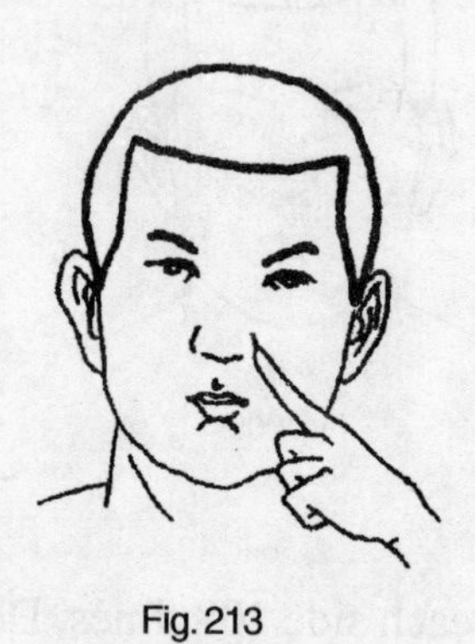

Fig. 213

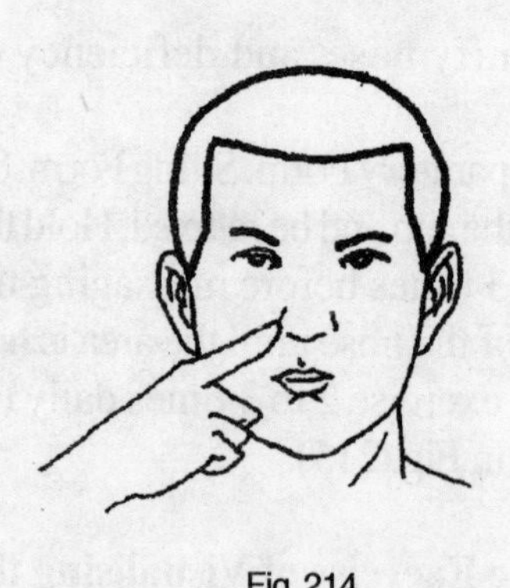

Fig. 214

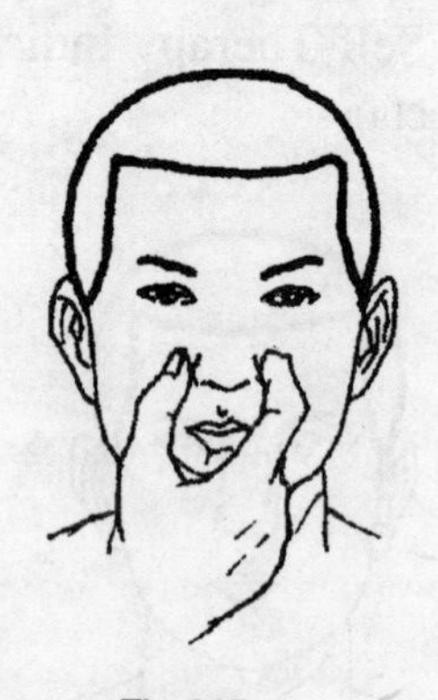

Fig. 215

Preparatory Form: Standing Form (2). Relax the whole body, keeping the mind on the acupoint of Fengfu (1.5 cun above the back hairline at the accipital part of the head, as shown in Fig. 216) for at least 20 minutes. Do the exercise every morning and evening.

18. The Exercise of Pressing Repeatedly the Acupoints of Erkuo

Self-Therapy Indication: Pain in the upper teeth.

Preparatory Form: Standing Form (2). Relax the whole body.

(1) Press repeatedly the acupoints of Erkuo in front of each auricle near the hairline at the upper side of the zygomatic region (as shown in Fig. 217) with the forefingers. Massage the acupoints clockwise 64 times and counterclockwise 64 times.

(2) Press hard the points about 5 cm below the acupoints of Quchi with the thumbs until you have a feeling of soreness and pain there (See Fig. 218).

19. The Exercise of Pressing Acupoints to Stop Pain

Self-Therapy Indication: Pain in the lower teeth.

Preparatory Form: Standing Form (2). Relax the whole body.

(1) Press hard the acupoints of Hegu (between the thumb and the forefinger at the back of the hand, a hollow between the first and the second metacarpal bones, as shown in Fig. 219) with your hands.

(2) Press hard and repeatedly the point 108 times in the chin (as shown in Fig. 220).

20. The Exercise of Channelling the Qi by the Mind

Self-Therapy Indication: Oral ulcer.

Preparatory Form: Standing Form (2). Relax the whole body, keeping your mind on the two acupoints of Jinjin and Yuye under the root of the tongue. Press hard on the two points under the

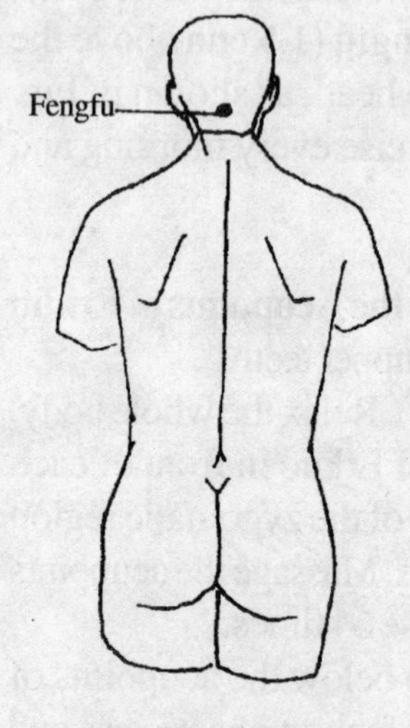

Fig. 216

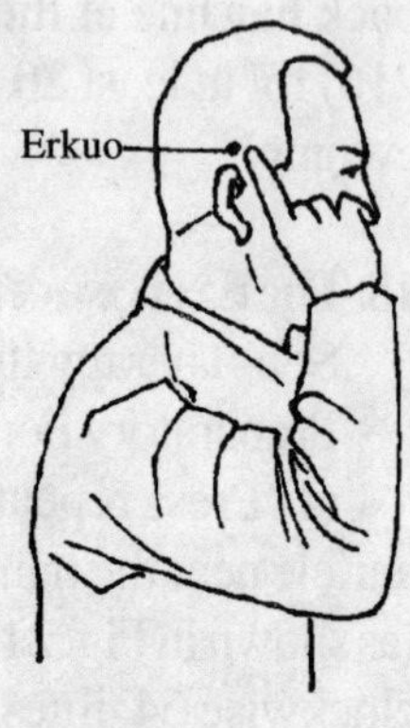

Fig. 217

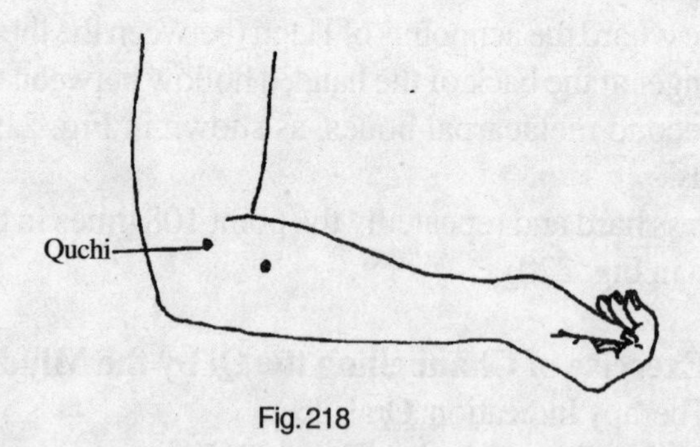

Fig. 218

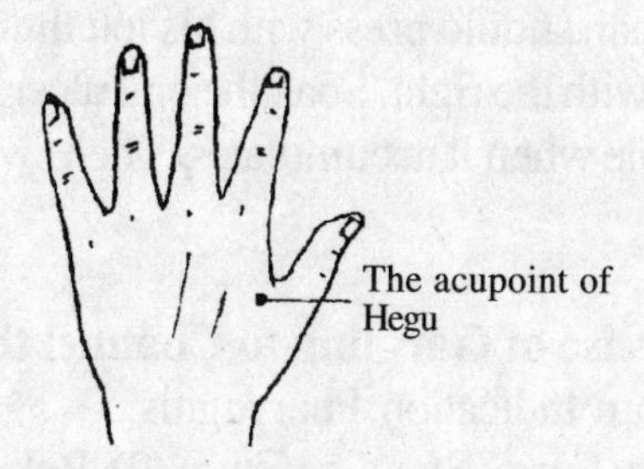

Fig. 219

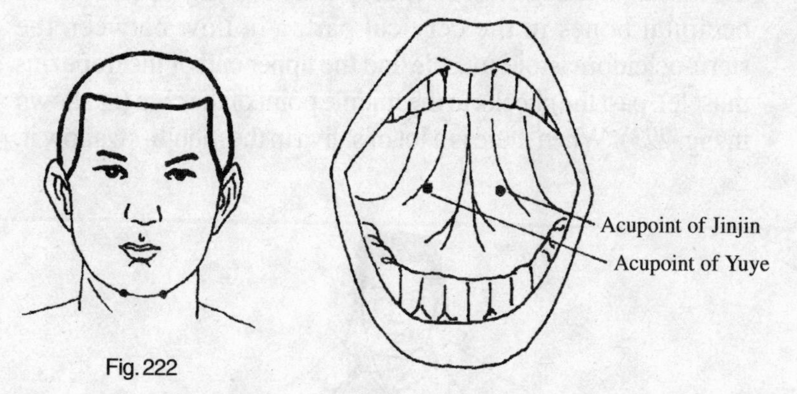

Fig. 222

Fig. 221

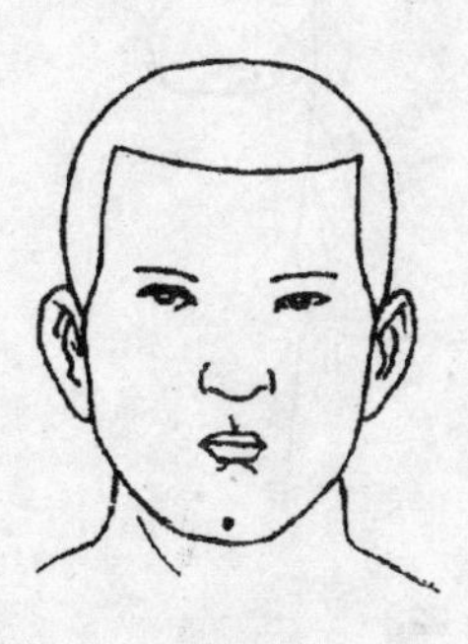

Fig. 220

corners of the mouth, at the lower side of the chin (as shown in Fig. 222). A man should press with his left thumb and forefinger and a woman with the right. Soak the oral ulcer in the saliva for as long as possible when it accumulates. Then swallow the saliva 3 times.

21. The Exercise of Gargling to Channel the Qi

Self-Therapy Indication: Pharyngitis.

Preparatory Form: Standing Form (2). Relax the whole body. Move your cheeks as if you are gargling. When there is saliva in the mouth, massage from the acupoints of Fengchi (below the occipital bones in the cervical part, a hollow between the stern-ocleidomastoid muscle and the upper end of the trapezius muscle), past the cheeks to the middle point of the chin (as shown in Fig. 223). When there is a lot of saliva in the mouth, swallow it.

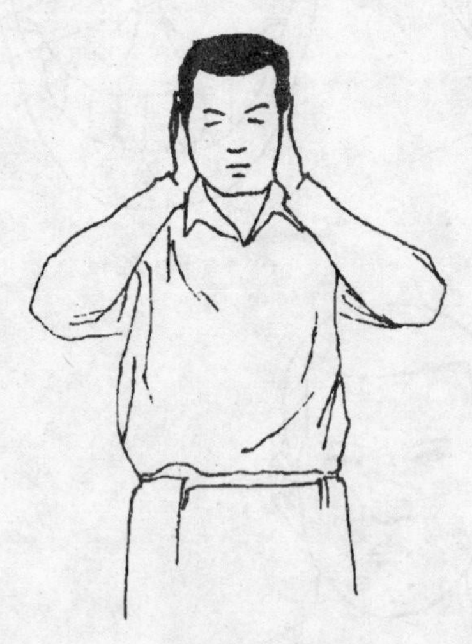

Fig. 223

Repeat the exercise 3 times.

Keep the tongue rolled up as far as possible, and swallow the saliva when there is any. Don't spit it out.

22. The Exercise of Pressing the Acupoints of Yinchi

Self-Therapy Indication: Hoarseness and laryngitis.

Preparatory Form: Sitting Form. Relax the whole body. Repeatedly press the acupoint of Yinchi (a point one cun away from the wrist's transverse line. There is one in each arm, as shown in Fig. 224) in the right arm with the left thumb 108 times, and the

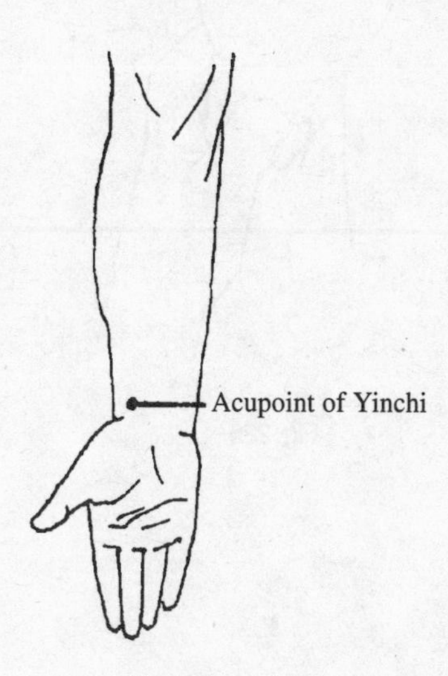

Fig. 224

acupoint of Yinchi in the left arm with the right thumb 108 times. Do the exercise every morning and evening (See Fig. 225).

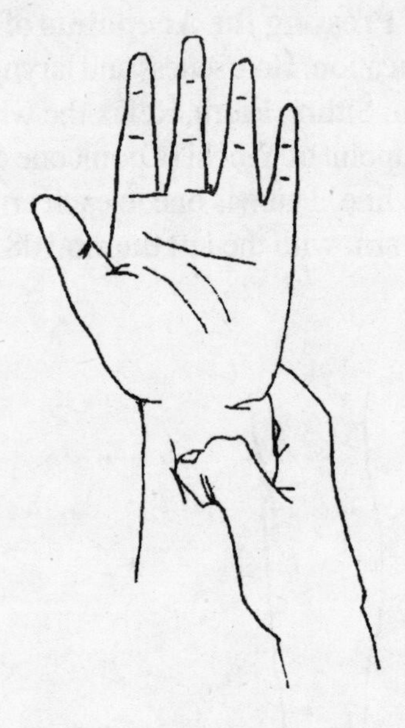

Fig. 225

CHAPTER X THE UROGENITAL SYSTEM

1. The Exercise of Crossing the Legs to Channel the Qi

Self-Therapy Indication: Difficulty of urination, and over frequent urination.

Preparatory Form: Sitting Form. Sit upright, keeping the whole body relaxed (as shown in Fig. 226). Keep your mind on the acupoint of Huiyin (a point between the anus and the root of the scrotum in males and between the anus and the posterior labial commissure in females), breathing naturally 24 times. Then raise the left leg and put it on the right thigh (as shown in Fig. 227). Then breathe deeply and gently 36 times before putting down the left leg. Raise the right leg and put it on the left thigh (as shown in Fig. 228), and then breath deeply and gently 36 times before putting down the right leg.

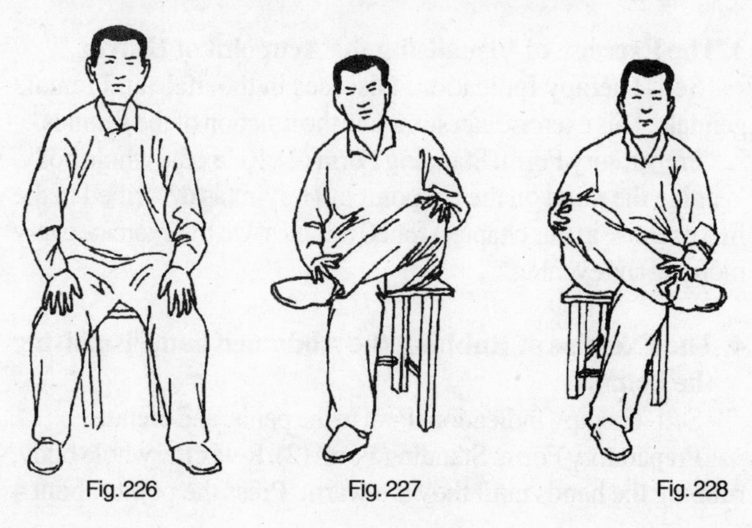

Fig. 226 Fig. 227 Fig. 228

2. The Exercise of Squatting to Channel the Qi

Self-Therapy Indication: Gonorrhoea and enuresis.

Squat down, leaning the trunk slightly forward. Move the hands past the outside of the thighs to the hollow of the knees, and then past the inside of the shanks to the insteps, holding the toes tightly and keeping them bent upward. If you can not reach the toes with your hands, hold the insteps and pull them inward until there is a little sweat all over the body. (See Fig. 229 and Fig. 230).

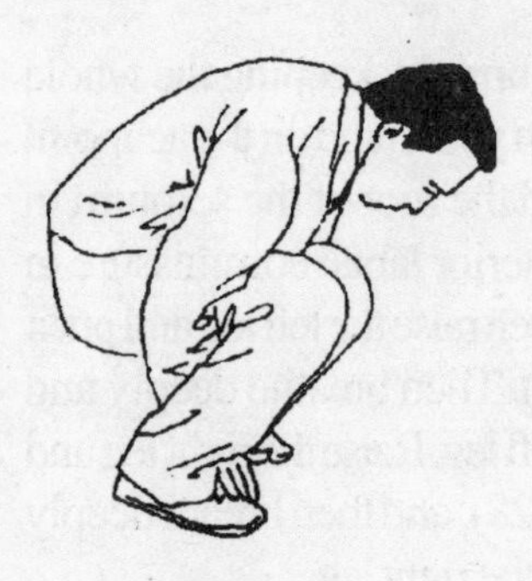

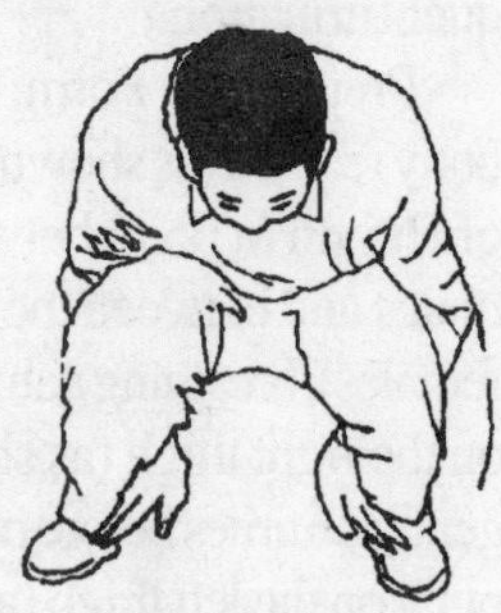

Fig. 230

Fig. 229

3. The Exercise of Visualising the Acupoint of Huiyin

Self-Therapy Indication: Diseases in the male and female genitals. This exercise can stimulate the function of the genitals.

Preparatory Form: Standing Form (2). Relax the whole body, keeping the mind on the acupoint of Huiyin (as described in the first exercise in this chapter) for 20 minutes. Do the exercise every morning and evening.

4. The Exercise of Rubbing the Abdomen and Visualising the Points

Self-Therapy Indication: Pain in the penis, and orchitis.

Preparatory Form: Standing Form (2). Relax the whole body, rubbing the hands until they are warm. Press the points about 4 cun below the navel, by the upper side of the groin with the acupoints of Inner Laogong (a point above the transverse line, between the second and the third metacarpal bones, where the middle finger tip touches when clenching a fist, as shown in Fig. 20). Rub the points up and down 64 times (as shown in Fig. 231).

Then relax the whole body, standing with the hands down. Visualise the points about 0.5 cun lateral to the acupoints of Guilai (4 cun below and 2 cun lateral to the navel. There is one on each side of the navel as shown in Fig. 232) for 20 minutes. Do the exercise before going to bed every night.

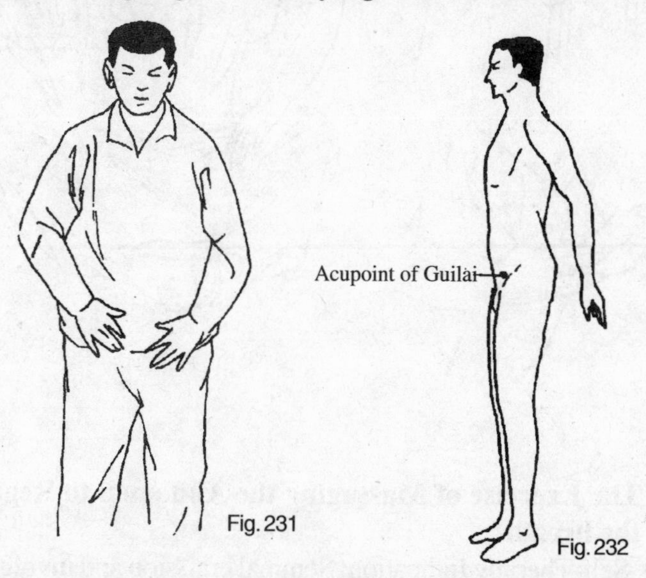

Fig. 231

Fig. 232

5. The Exercise of Rubbing and Brushing the Legs and the Feet

Self-Therapy Indication: Impotence, and the decline of sexual functions.

Sit on a chair or an armchair. Rub the two soles of the feet 108 times respectively (as shown in Fig. 233). Sit down with your soles touching each other, keeping your knees outward. Brush the thighs from the inside of the knees up to the groin. Brush the left and the right thighs 108 times respectively (as shown in Fig. 234). Do the exercise before going to bed.

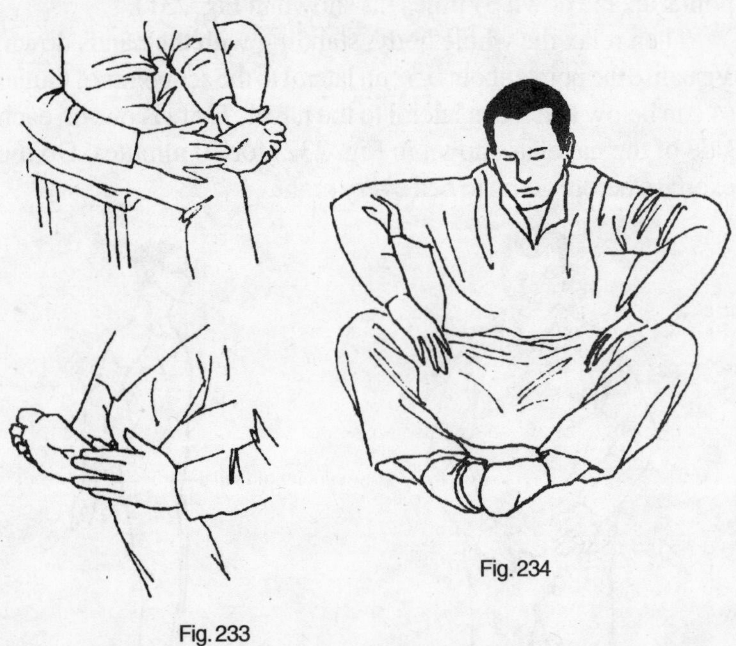
Fig. 234

Fig. 233

6. The Exercise of Massaging the Abdomen to Regulate the Breath

Self-Therapy Indication: Seminal emission and involuntary emissions.

Preparatory Form: Standing Form (2). Relax the whole body. Press the abdomen hard with two hands, with the right palm on top of the left hand. Make 36 clockwise rotations with the overlapped hands and 36 counterclockwise rotations (as shown in Fig. 235). Inhale the air slowly, imagining it is flowing to the acupoint of Mingmen (a point in a hollow below the spinous process of the second lumbar vertebra, as shown in Fig. 57) while clenching fists tightly, drawing the lower abdomen in and the anus up before exhaling slowly. Breathe in this way 7 times before concluding. Lie on your side and bend your knees when sleeping (as shown in Fig. 236). To persist in doing this exercise before going to bed preserves the semen.

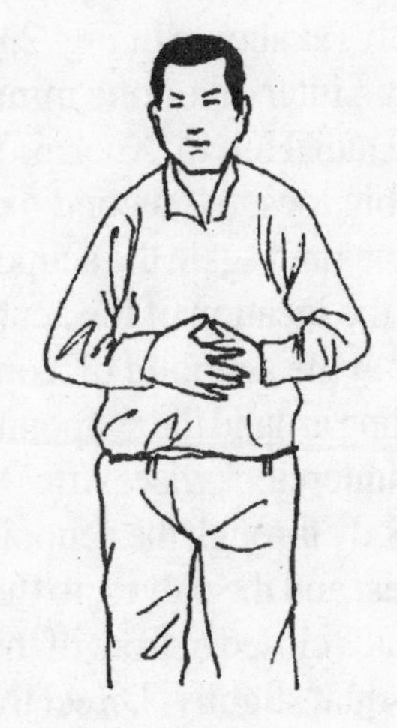

Fig. 235

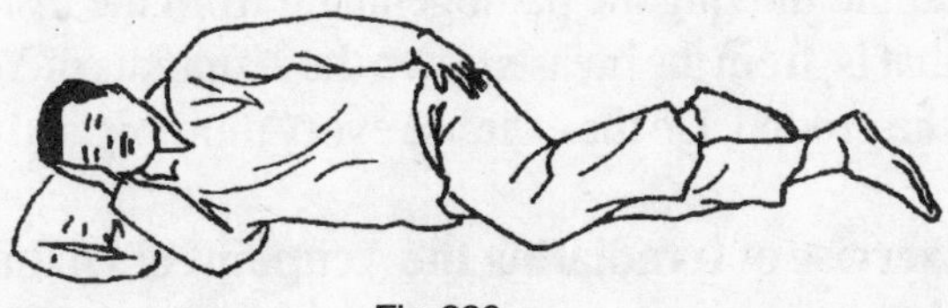

Fig. 236

CHAPTER XI GYNECOLOGICAL SYSTEM

1. The Exercise of Irradiating the Breasts with the Qi

Self-Therapy Indication: Mastitis.

Preparatory Form: Standing Form (2). Relax the whole body, closing the eyes gently (as shown in Fig. 237). Visualise the following acupoints at an interval of one minute or a half: Baihui, Jianjing, Danzhong, Duqi, Huiyin, Xuehai, Yinlingquan, Sanyinjiao, Yongquan, the big toes, the second toes, the third toes, the fourth toes, the little toes and again the acupoints of Yongquan (as shown in Fig. 25 for the location of the acupoints). Imagine that there is a mass of air at the acupoint of Yongquan in the sole of each foot, the air circling around the acupoint 36 times clockwise, and then 36 times counterclockwise. After that, imagine that the air comes into your body through the acupoints of Yongquan and flows along the ankles, and the calves, to the lower abdomen.

Stand with the hands closed in front of the chest for 5 minutes. Bend the knees and squat slightly. Direct the palms to the lower part of each breast, the distance apart being 10 cm. Stand 10 more minutes. You will feel hot in the breasts (as shown in Fig. 238). Imagine moving the pathogenic Qi from the inside to the outside, that is, from the breasts down the acupoints of Yongquan and into the ground. Do the exercise every morning and evening.

2. The Exercise of Irradiating the Acupoint of Qizhong with the Qi

Self-Therapy Indication: Deficiency of the blood of a female, and asthma.

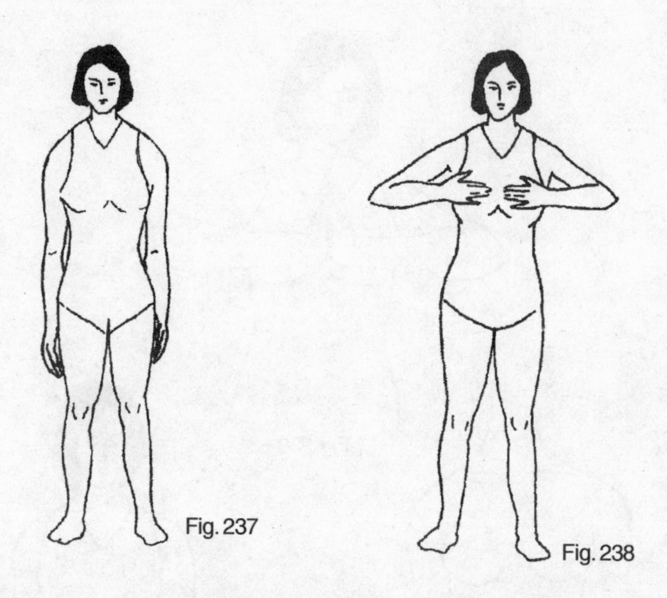
Fig. 237
Fig. 238

Preparatory Form: Standing Form (2). Relax the whole body, stretching the arms to the left and right. Move them in an arc upward and forward, the hands closed in front of the chest. Bend the knees slightly, looking at the middle fingers (as shown in Fig. 239). After 10 minutes, separate the hands and direct the acupoints of Laogong (a point above the transverse line, between the second and the third metacarpal bones, where the middle finger tip touches when clenching a fist, as shown in Fig. 20) to the acupoints of Qizhong (1.5 cun below and lateral to the navel, on both sides of it, as shown in Fig. 240). The distance apart should be about 10 cm (as shown in Fig. 241). Stand for 10 to 20 minutes each time. Do the exercise every morning and evening.

3. The Exercise of Moxibustion at the Acupoints of Guanyi

Self-Therapy Indication: Pain in the lower abdomen of a female, and pain in the female's pudendum.

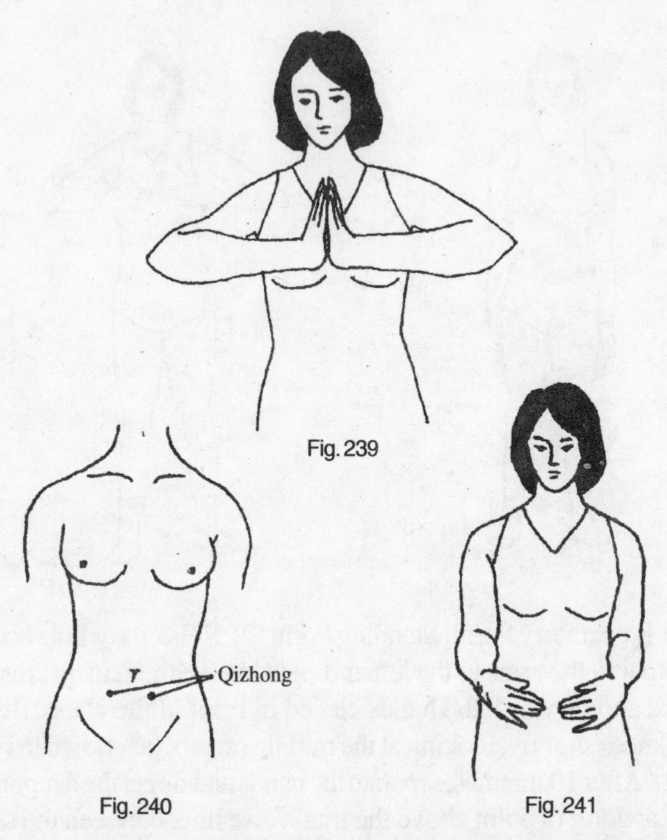

Fig. 239

Fig. 240

Fig. 241

Lie on the stomach on a bed. Administer moxibustion at the acupoints of Guanyi (in the hollow one cun above the transverse line of the knee hollow, at both legs as shown in Fig. 242 and Fig. 243) with moxarolls for 10 minutes. Administer the moxibustion every morning and evening.

4. The Exercise of Massaging the Abdomen and Regulating the Breath

Self-Therapy Indication: Diseases in a female's genitals.

Both the standing and sitting forms will do.

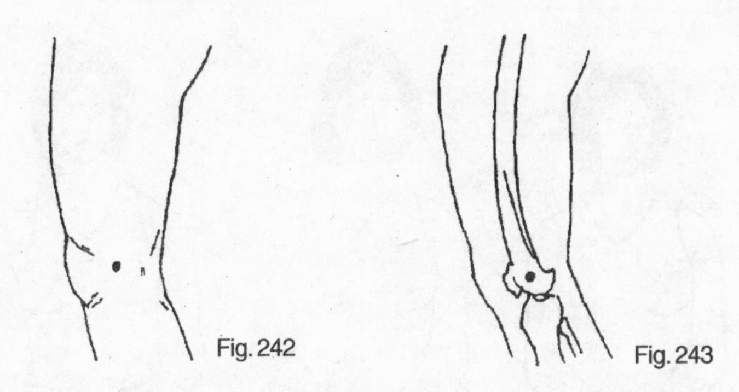
Fig. 242 Fig. 243

Preparatory Form: Standing Form (2). Let the hands hang down naturally. Press the lower abdomen with the right palm, the left palm on top of the right hand (as shown in Fig. 244). Imagine there is a ball inside the lower abdomen that makes 36 clockwise rotations under the hands, and 36 counterclockwise rotations after that.

Deep breathing exercise: Imagine that the navel is pressing at the acupoint of Mingmen (in the hollow below the spinous process of the second lumbar vertebra, as shown in Fig. 57). Exhale naturally. Breathe 36 times.

The exercises in the sitting form are the same as those in the standing form. Do the exercise every morning and evening.

5. The Exercise of Rubbing and Irradiating the Abdomen

Self-Therapy Indication: Menorrhagia, and excessive leukorrhea.

Preparetory Form: Standing Form (2). Press the lower abdomen with the right palm, with the left palm on top of the right hand (as shown in Fig. 245). Make 36 clockwise circles on the lower abdomen with the hands and 36 counterclockwise circles.

Preparatory Form: Standing Form (2). Bend the knees slightly, rubbing the hands 108 times. Keep your mind on the palms. Keep

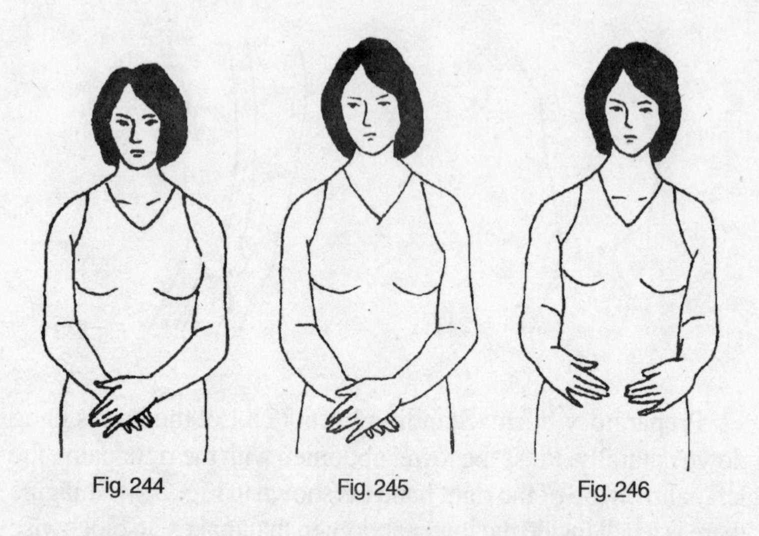
Fig. 244 Fig. 245 Fig. 246

your hands in front of the lower abdomen, with all the fingers pointing to each other, the distance between the fingers being 5 cm, and the distance between the hands and the lower abdomen being 10 cm. Irradiate the lower abdomen with the palms (as shown in Fig. 246) and at the same time keep your mind on the acupoint of Dantian (as shown in Fig. 37) and imagine the acupoint being warm and you will begin to feel hot of this point. Stand for 10 to 15 minutes.

6. The Exercise of Moxibustion at the Acupoints of Shiguan

Self-Therapy Indication: Acute postpartum pain in the legs.

Both the standing and sitting forms will do. Administer moxibustion at the acupoints of Shiguan (4 cuns below and 1 cun lateral to the nipples of the breasts, as shown in Fig. 247) with moxarolls for 10 minutes, and for 10 more minutes if the pain is not relieved.

7. The Exercise of Irradiating the Acupoints of Bailao

Self -Therapy Indication: Postpartum pain all over the body.

Preparatory Form: Standing Form (2). Relax the whole body. Rub the hands until they are warm. Rub the acupoints of Bailao (at the back of the neck, one cun below the hairline and one cun lateral to the center of the neck, as shown in Fig. 248.) up and down 108 times with the palms. Press the root of the palms to the hairline, with the acupoints of Laogong (above the transverse line, between the second and the third metacarpal bones, where the middle finger tip touches when clenching a fist, as shown in Fig. 20) against the acupoints of Bailao. Keep the distance between the acupoints of Laogong and Bailao 3 to 5 cm from each other, irradiating the acupoints of Bailao with Qi for 10 minutes.

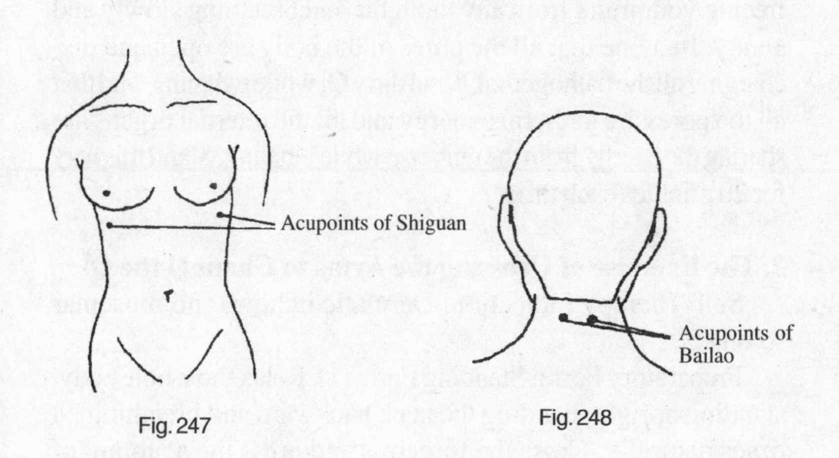

Fig. 247

Fig. 248

CHAPTER XII SURGICAL SYSTEM

1. The Exercise of Regulating the Breath Through the Pores

Self-Therapy Indication: Dermatoses.

Preparatory Form: Standing Form (2). Relax the whole body, keeping the eyes nearly closed or looking forwards, but without seeing anything. Bend the knees slightly (as shown in Fig. 249), freeing your mind from any thoughts and breathing slowly and gently. Imagine that all the pores of the body are open and discharging all the pathogenic Qi and dirty Qi while exhaling, and that all the pores are gathering energy and all the internal organs are sharing the energy from the universe while inhaling. Stand this way for 20 minutes each time.

2. The Exercise of Crossing the Arms to Channel the Qi

Self-Therapy Indication: Dermatic itching, and muscular spasms.

Preparatory Form: Standing Form (1). Relax the whole body, standing upright, bending the neck backward and breathing 24 times naturally. Cross the forearms and press the acupoint of right Jianjing (a mid-point between the spinous process of the seventh cervical vertebra and the acromin, at the acromial extremity of clavide, as shown in Fig. 134) with the left hand, and the acupoint of left Jianjing with the right hand (as shown in Fig. 250). Don't move the hands, but raise the elbows higher than the shoulders. Move the elbows up and down 24 times (as shown in Fig. 251).

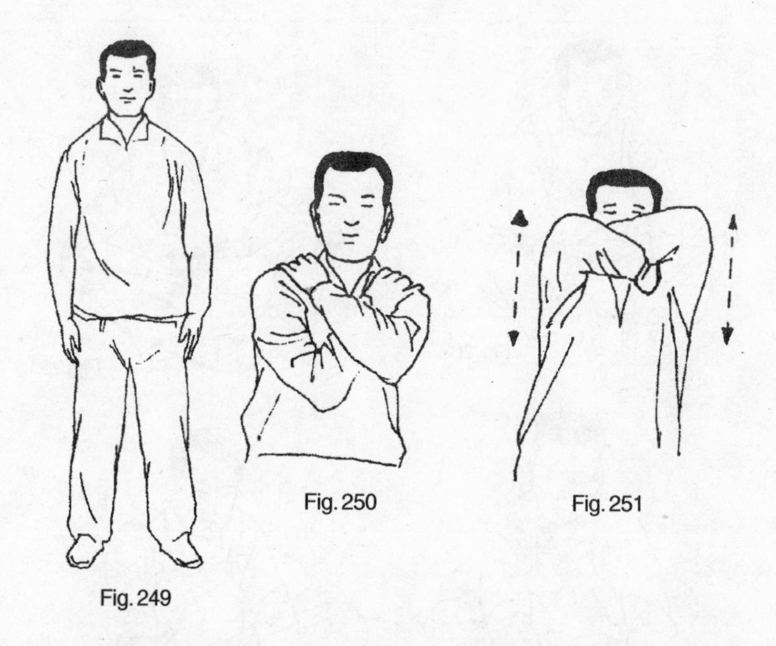

Fig. 249 Fig. 250 Fig. 251

3. The Exercise of Sitting and Grasping the Feet

Self-Therapy Indication: Piles, pain and cold in the knees.

Sit upright on a bed, bending the knees outward, with the two soles of your feet touching each other. Hold the feet with the hands and pull them toward the arms (as shown in Fig. 252). Then pull the knees upward with the hands without separating the feet (as shown in Fig. 253). After that, be relaxed and lower the knees naturally, returning to the former position. Pull the knees upward 24 times. Grasp the feet, the trunk making 24 clockwise rotations and 24 counterclockwise rotations (as shown in Fig. 254 and Fig. 255).

4. The Exercise of Pressing the Acupoints of Dingshu

Self-Therapy Indication: Furuncle and carbuncle.

Preparatory Form: Sitting Form (1). Relax the whole body.

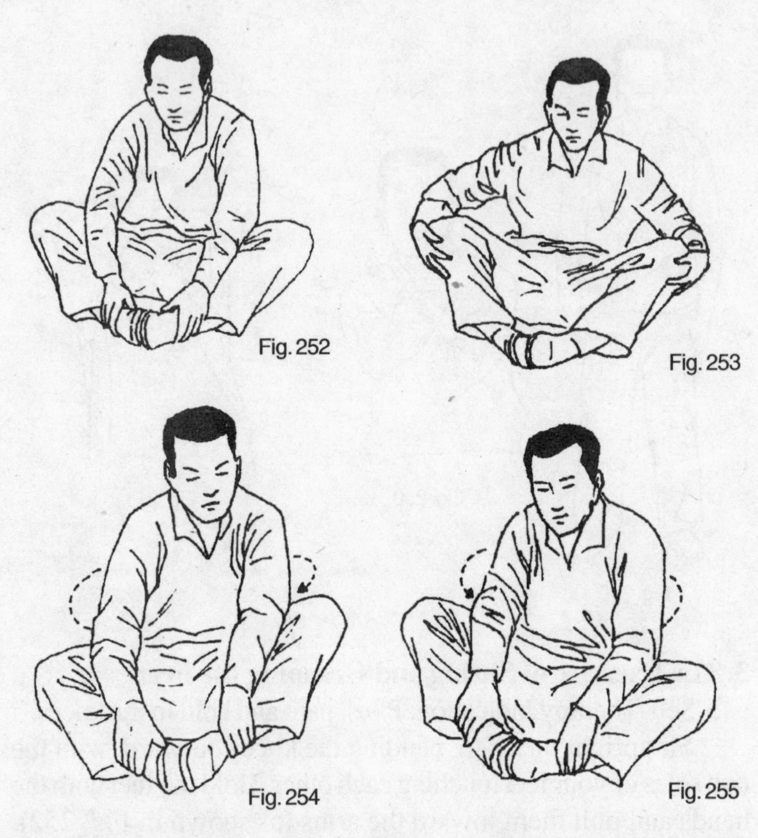
Fig. 252
Fig. 253
Fig. 254
Fig. 255

Repeatedly press the acupoint of Dingshu (a point 4 cun above the third transverse line of the wrist. There is one in each arm, as shown in Fig. 256) in the right forearm 108 times with the left thumb. Then press repeatedly the acupoint of Dingshu in the left arm 108 times with the right thumb (as shown in Fig. 257). Do the exercise every morning and evening.

5. The Exercise for Channelling the Qi Through the Body

Self-Therapy Indication: Hernia, a mass in a female's abdomen, stimulating the circulation of the blood.

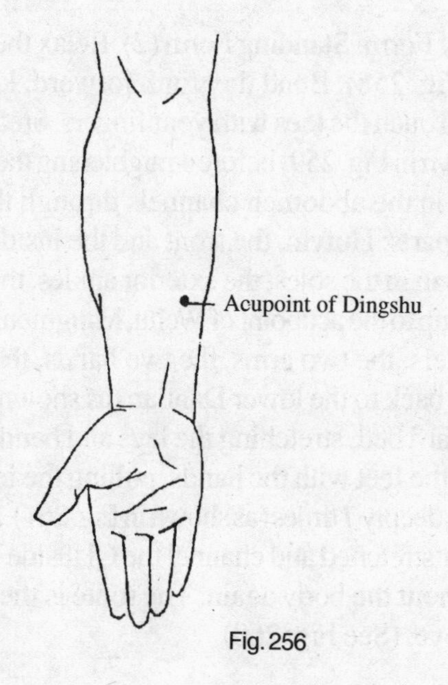

Fig. 256

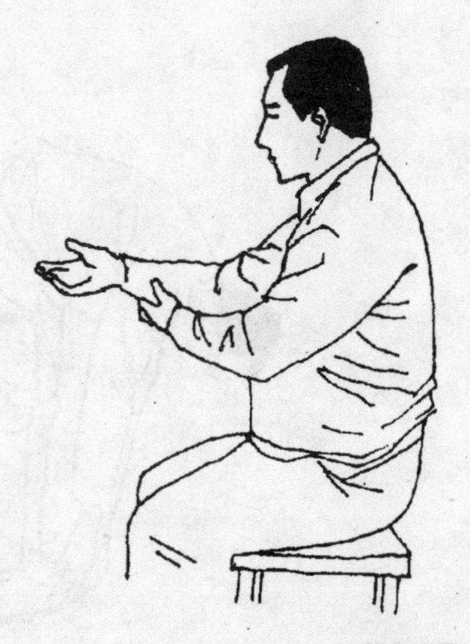
Fig. 257

Preparatory Form: Standing Form (2). Relax the whole body (as shown in Fig. 258). Bend the trunk forward, keep the knee joints straight. Touch the toes with your fingers, breathing deeply 7 times (as shown in Fig. 259) before straightening the trunk. Imagine that the Qi in the abdomen channels through the following acupoints and parts: Huiyin, the front and the inside parts of the thighs, Yongquan in the soles, the exterior ankles, the outside and rear of the legs, up to the acupoint of Weilu, Mingmen, Jiaji, Baihui, the two shoulders, the two arms, the two hands, the acupoint of Danzhong and back to the lower Dantian (as shown in Fig. 260). Then sit on a hard bed, stretching the legs and bending the trunk forward. Hold the feet with the hands, pulling the feet backward while breathing deeply 7 times (as shown in Fig. 261). Sit up straight with the feet outstretched and channel the Qi inside the lower abdomen throughout the body again. The route is the same as that mentioned above. (See Fig. 260)

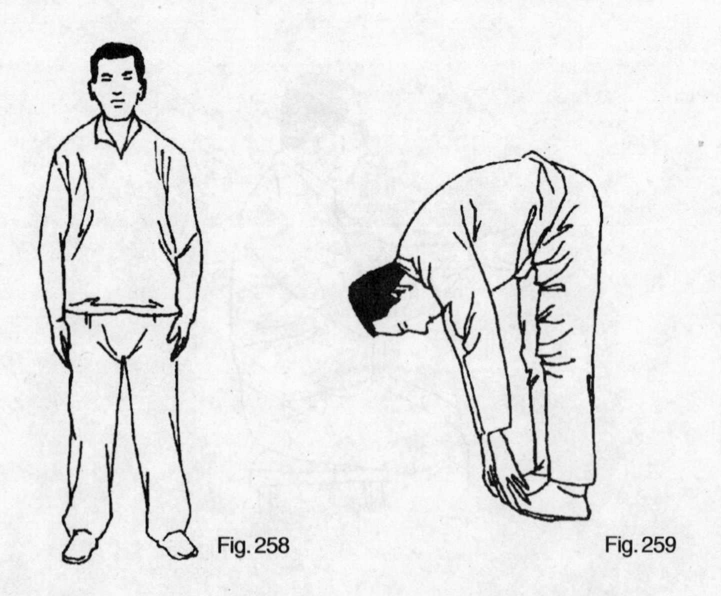

Fig. 258

Fig. 259

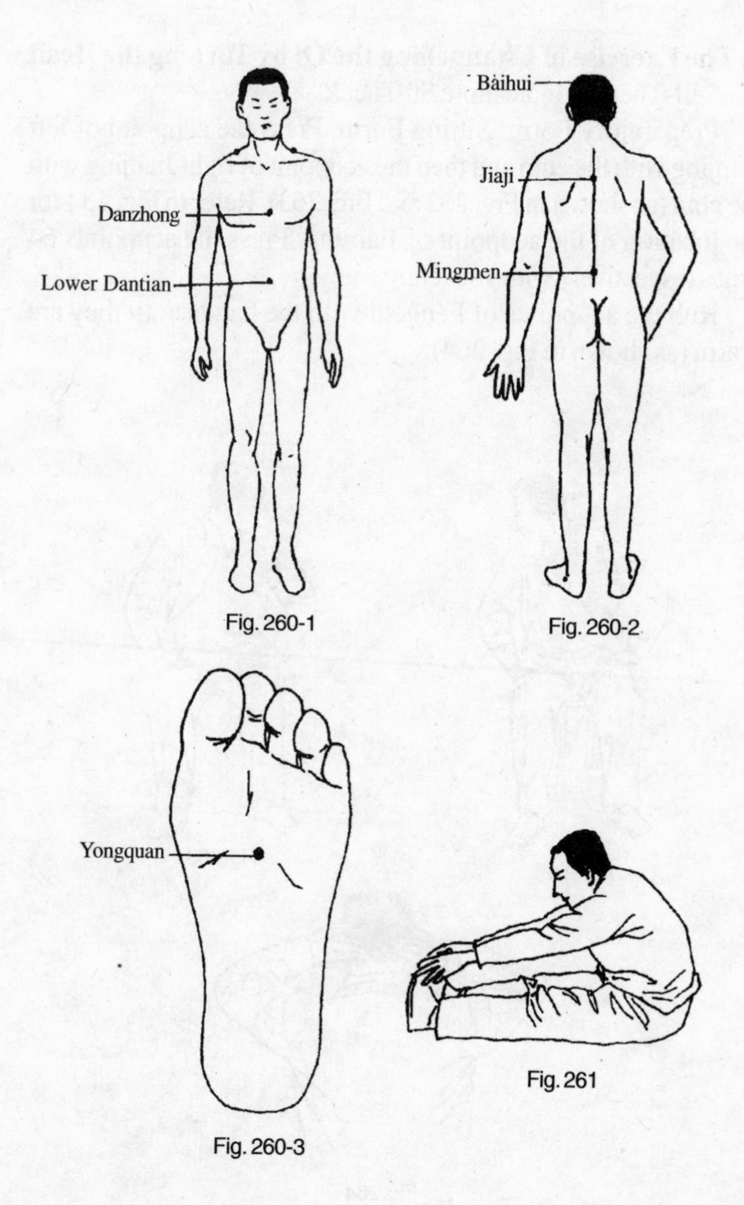

Fig. 260-1

Fig. 260-2

Fig. 260-3

Fig. 261

6. The Exercise of Channelling the Qi by Turning the Head

Self-Therapy Indication: Stiff neck.

Preparatory Form: Sitting Form. Press the acupoint of left Jianjing with the chin and then the acupoint of right Jianjing with the chin (as shown in Fig. 262 and Fig. 263). Refer to Fig. 134 for the location of the acupoint of Jianjing. Press the acupoints 64 times respectively with your chin.

Rub the acupoints of Fengchi with the hands until they are warm (as shown in Fig. 264).

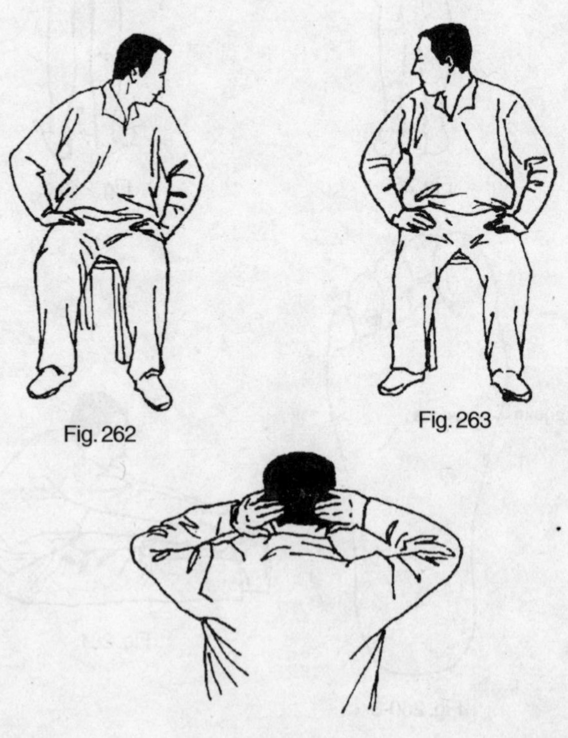

Fig. 262

Fig. 263

Fig. 264

7. The Exercise of Lying on the Side to Channel the Qi

Self-Therapy Indication: Chronic appendicitis.

Preparatory Form: Standing Form (2). Relax the whole body, with the hands closed in front of the chest (as shown in Fig. 265) for 5 minutes. Then press the points about 4 cun below and 3 cun lateral to the navel with the acupoints of Laogong (above the transverse line, between the second and the third metacarpal bones, where the middle finger tip touches when clenching a fist, refer to Fig. 20), (as shown in Fig. 266). After 5 minutes, massage the two points inward and downword 36 times and 36 times in the opposite direction. Continue thereafter to press the points for 5 minutes with the hands.

8. The Exercise of Visualising the Acupoints of Lanwei

Self-Therapy Indication: Acute appendicitis.

Preparatory Form: Sitting Form. Relax the whole body. Press repeatedly the acupoints of Lanwei (in the calves' fibular, 5.5 cun

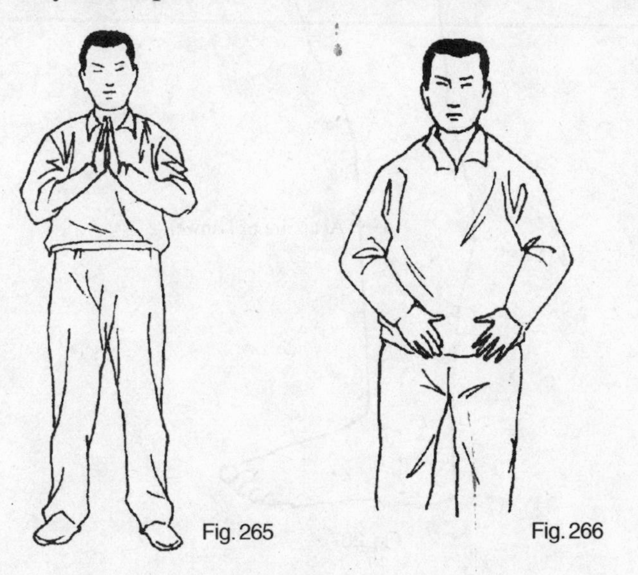

Fig. 265 Fig. 266

right below the knee caps, outside the anterior tibia muscle, as shown in Fig. 267) with the thumb, pressing hard and you will have a feeling of soreness and distension in the insteps. Then relax the whole body, closing the eyes and visualising the acupoints of Lanwei for 20 minutes.

9. The Exercise of Breathing Through the Acupoint of Dantian

Self-Therapy Indication: Piles and prostatitis.

Preparatory Form: Sitting Form. Attach the acupoint of Laogong in the left hand (above the transverse line, between the second and the third metacarpal bones, where the middle finger tip touches when clenching a fist, as shown in Fig. 20) to the navel with the acupoint of Laogong in the right palm on top of the acupoint of Outer Laogong (at the back of the hand as shown in Fig. 268)

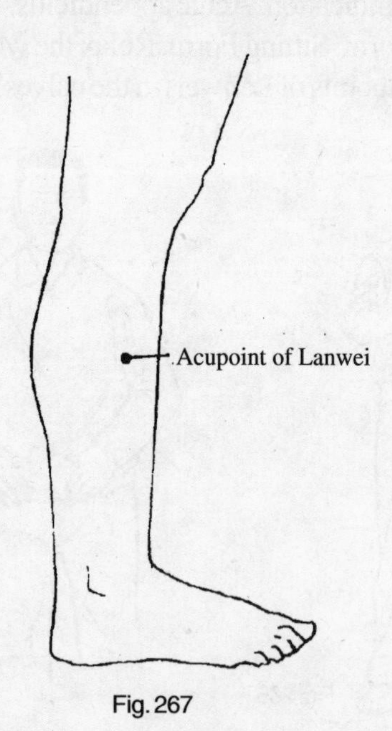

Fig. 267

in the left hand. Draw the lower abdomen in while inhaling. Imagine the lower abdomen as touching the acupoint of Mingmen in a hollow below the spinous process of the second lumbar vertebra, as shown in Fig. 57). Pull the anus up. Imagine attaching the acupoint of Mingmen to the navel when exhaling. Breathe 108 times. Then return to the former sitting form (as shown in Fig. 269).

10. The Exercise of Channelling the Qi Through the Acupoint of Huiyin

Self-Therapy Indication: Scrotum eczema.

Standing naturally, feet apart, holding the testis with the left hand. Massage the lower part of the testis with the right hand. Pull and push it 64 times. Do the exercise every morning and evening.

11. The Exercise of Visualising the Acupoints of Chongmen

Self-Therapy Indication: Hernia, difficulty in urination.

Preparatory Form: Standing Form (2). Relax the whole body.

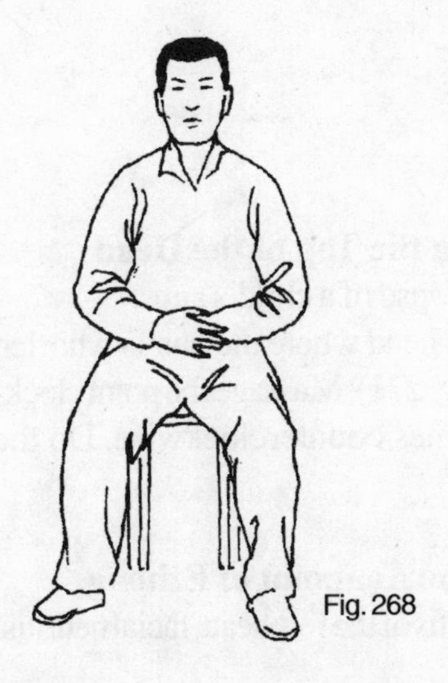

Fig. 268

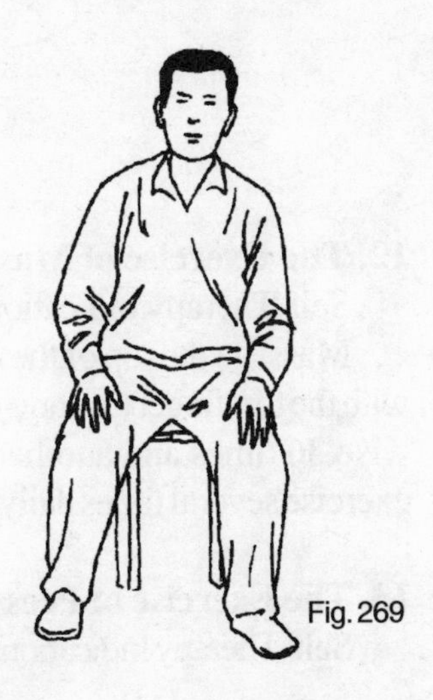

Fig. 269

Visualise the acupoints of Chongmen at the upper end of each groin and outside the femoral artery (as shown in Fig. 270). Stand for at least 20 minutes each time. Do the exercise every morning and evening.

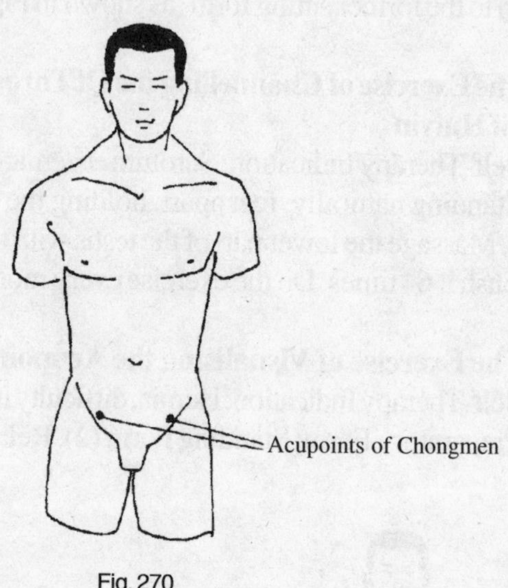

Fig. 270

12. The Exercise of Massaging the Top of the Head

Self-Therapy Indication: Prolapse of a child's anus.

Massage the top of the child's head where the hair is whorled with the forefinger (as shown in Fig. 271). Massage the point clockwise 36 times and another 36 times counterclockwise. Do the exercise several times daily.

13. The Exercise of Pressing the Acupoint of Ezhong

Self-Therapy Indication: Sinustis of the forehead, facial neuritis.

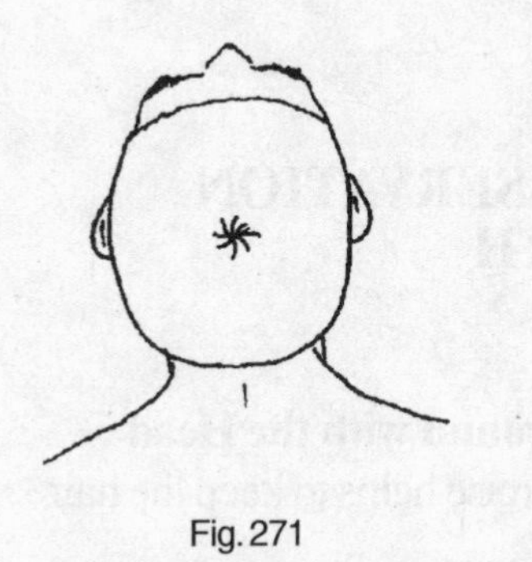
Fig. 271

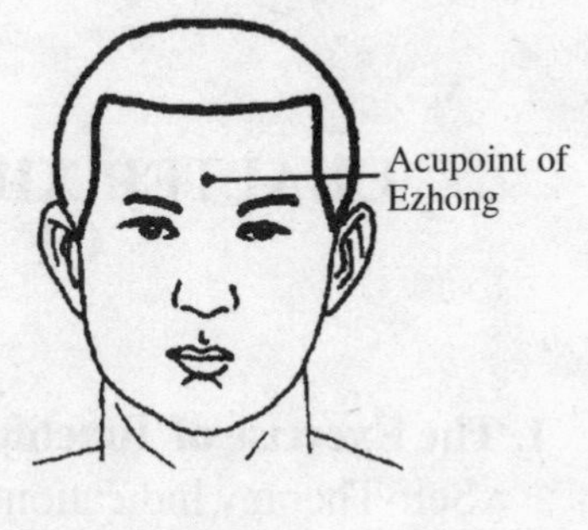

Fig. 272

Preparatory Form: Sitting Form. Relax the whole body. Press repeatedly the acupoint of Ezhong (the middle line of the forhead, one third of the distance between the eyebrows and the front hair line, as shown in Fig. 272) 108 times with the middle fingers. Do the exercise every morning and evening.

CHAPTER XIII PRESERVATION OF HEALTH

1. The Exercise of Touching the Ground with the Head

Self-Therapy Indication: This exercise helps to keep the hair soft, smooth and in good condition.

Sit upright on a hard bed, stretching your legs and relaxing your whole body. Put the hands on the knees (as shown in Fig. 273). Bend the trunk forward as far as possible, keeping the head close to the shanks (as shown in Fig. 274). When your head can touch the shanks easily, after a period of practise, separate the feet about 33 cm apart, putting the hands on the shanks and bending the trunk forward to make your head touch the bed (as shown in Fig. 275). Repeat the exercise 24 times.

2. The Exercise of Combing the Hair and Pressing Acupoints

Self-Therapy Indication: Trichomadesis.

Preparatory Form: Standing Form (2). Look straight forward. Relax the shoulders and the elbows, stretching the arms to the left and right. Move the hands upward and forward in an arc, the hands closed in front of the chest and the two acupoints of Inner Laogong (above the transverse line, between the second and the third metacarpal bones, where the middle finger tip touches when clenching a fist as shown in Fig. 20) touching each other without exerting force. Keep your mind on the centre of the palms for 5 minutes (as shown in Fig. 276).

Comb the hair 108 times with the fingers. It is desirable to keep combing until you feel a little pain in your scalp. Press re-

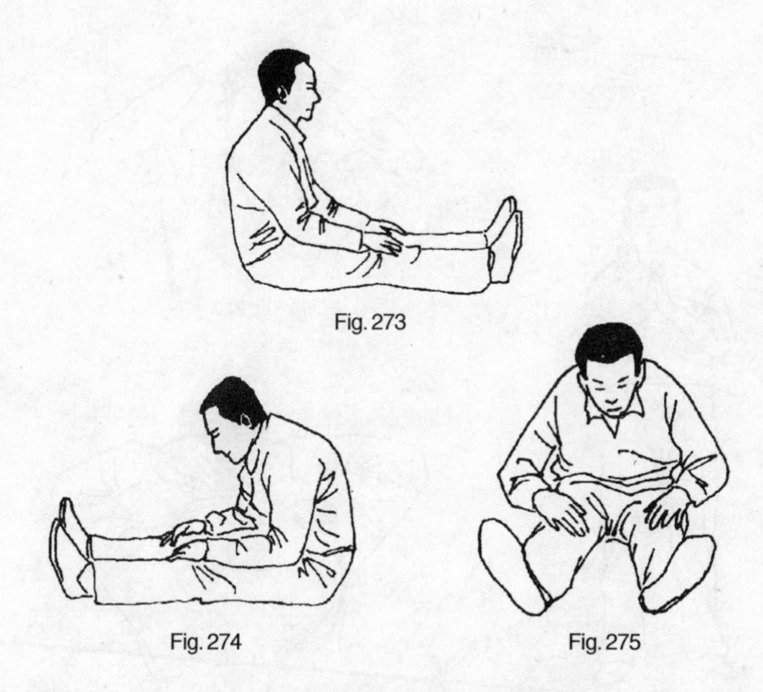
Fig. 273

Fig. 274

Fig. 275

peatedly the acupoint of Baihui (at the center of the top of the head, as shown in Fig. 33.) 36 times with two forefingers (as shown in Fig. 277).

Rub the acupoint of Fengchi up and down 36 times (as shown in Fig. 278).

3. The Exercise of Massaging the Teeth

Self-Therapy Indication: Periodontitis, keeping an elderly person's teeth in good condition.

Wash your hands before inserting your left forefinger into your mouth to massage the right upper and lower gum 36 times respectively. Then insert the right forefinger into your mouth, massaging the left upper and lower gum 36 times respectively (as shown in Fig. 279 and Fig. 280). Before massaging the gum, spread a

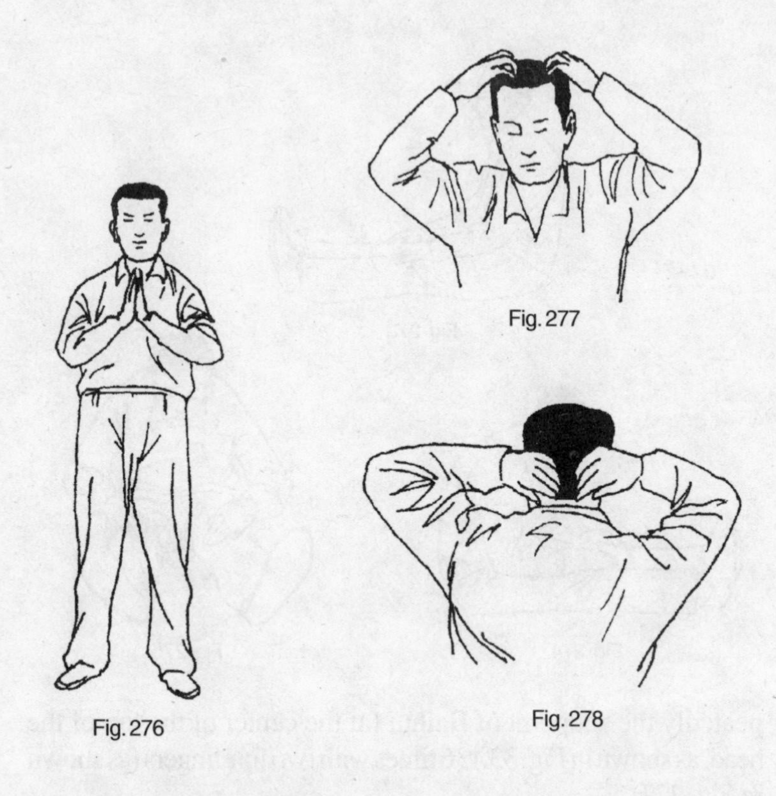
Fig. 276
Fig. 277
Fig. 278

little salt on the finger cushion, and gargle with water after massaging. Stop applying salt when the gum doesn't bleed.

Massaging the gum frequently can keep the gum full and round, and the teeth tough.

4. The Exercise for Prolonging Life by Using Moxibustion

Self-Therapy Indication: In the Chinese lunar calendar there are 24 divisions, called solar terms, in a solar year. When the solar terms change from one to another, the temperature changes and people are liable to chronic diseases, especially the elderly persons aged and invalids. On the day beginning a new solar term,

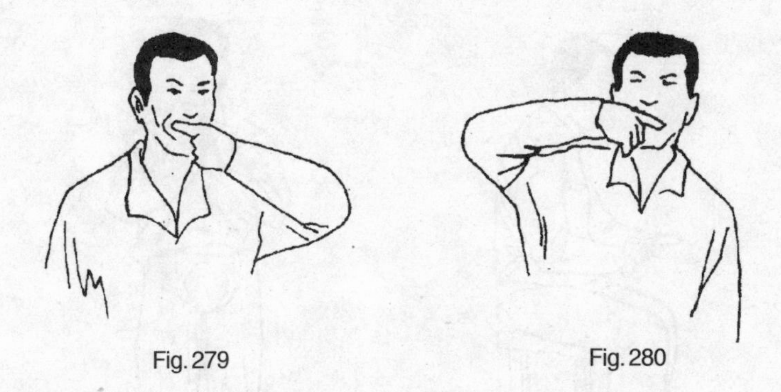
Fig. 279　　Fig. 280

either in the morning or evening of that day, administer moxibustion at the abdomen with a moxaroll. The exercise can prevent an attack of chronic disease, keep you fit and prolong your life.

Preparatory Form: Sitting Form. When it is the first day of the Spring Equinox (the 4th solar term, March 20 or 21), the Autumnal Equinox (the 16th solar term, September. 22, 23 or 24), the Winter Solstice (the 22nd solar term, December. 21, 22 or 23), and the Summer Solstice (the 10th solar term, June 21 or 22), get a moxaroll, which can be bought at a Chinese medicine shop and light it, holding it near the navel at a distance of 3 to 5 cm. When you feel hot in the navel, move the moxaroll a little farther away. Each moxibustion should last for 20 minutes (as shown in Fig. 281).

5. The Exercise for the Circulation of the Qi Ending at the Acupoint of Dantian

Self-Therapy Indication: This exercise can regulate the balance of *Yin* and *Yang* in the body, and make the metabolism exuberant.

Preparatory Form: Standing Form (2). Relax the whole body, and close the eyes gently, with the hands closed in front of the

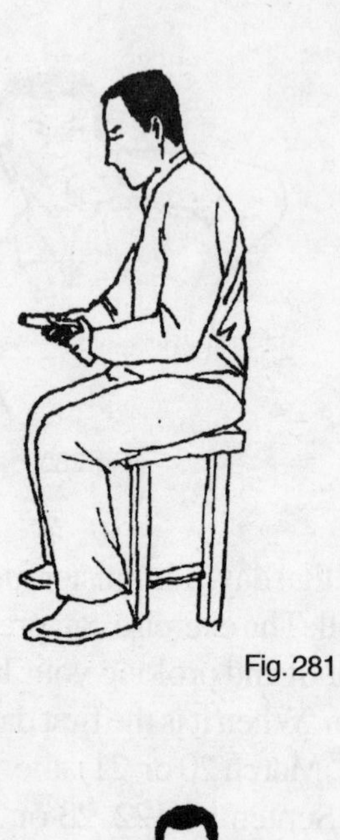

Fig. 281

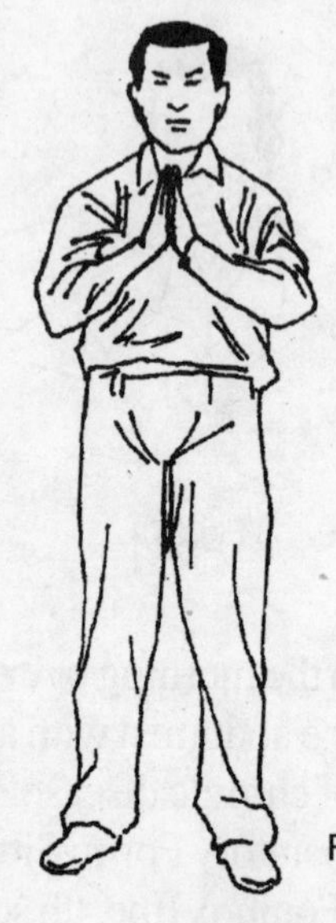

Fig. 282

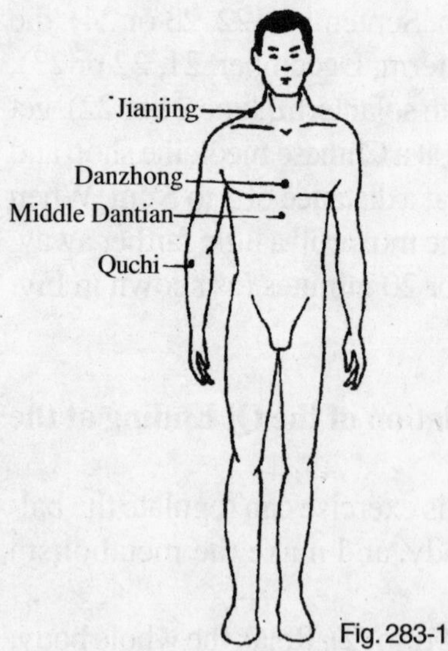

Fig. 283-1

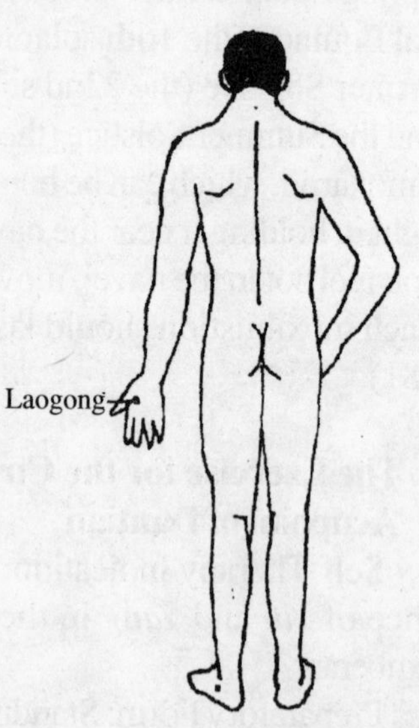

Fig. 283-2

chest (as shown in Fig. 282). Visualise the acupoint of Middle Dantian first, and then the acupoint of Danzhong, the acupoint of left Jianjing, the acupoint of left Quchi, the acupoint of left Outer Laogong, the left middle finger tip, the acupoint of left Inner Laogong, and then the acupoint right Inner Laogong, the right middle finger tip, the acupoint of right Outer Laogong, the acupoint of right Quchi, the acupoint of right Jianjing, the acupoint of Danzhong, and finally end the cycle at the acupoint of Middle Dantian. Repeat the exercise 3 times (as shown in Fig. 283).

图书在版编目（CIP）数据
常见病自己治：英文/李和生编著.
－北京：外文出版社，2001
ISBN 7-119-02061-7
I. 常… II. 李… Ⅲ.常见病－疗法－普及读物—英文
IV. R45-49
中国版本图书馆 CIP 数据核字（97）第 10123 号

责任编辑　杨春燕
英文编辑　许　荣
封面设计　唐少文
插图绘制　程星涛
印刷监制　张国祥

外文出版社网址:
http://www.flp.com.cn
外文出版社电子信箱:
info@flp.com.cn
sales@flp.com.cn

常见病自己治
李和生　编著
*

外文出版社出版
(中国北京百万庄大街 24 号)
邮政编码　100037
汇鑫印务有限公司印刷
中国国际图书贸易总公司发行
(中国北京车公庄西路 35 号)
北京邮政信箱第 399 号　邮政编码　100044
2001 年(大 32 开)第 1 版
2006 年第 1 版第 2 次印刷
(英)
ISBN 7-119-02061-7/R.158(外)
03000(平)
14-E-3212 P